Code Green

How the Big Lie in Healthcare Affects Us All

JOHN A. KELLUM M.D.

PAGE PUBLISHING
Conneaut Lake, PA

First originally published by Page Publishing 2024

ISBN 979-8-89315-139-8 (pbk)
ISBN 979-8-89315-151-0 (digital)

Printed in the United States of America

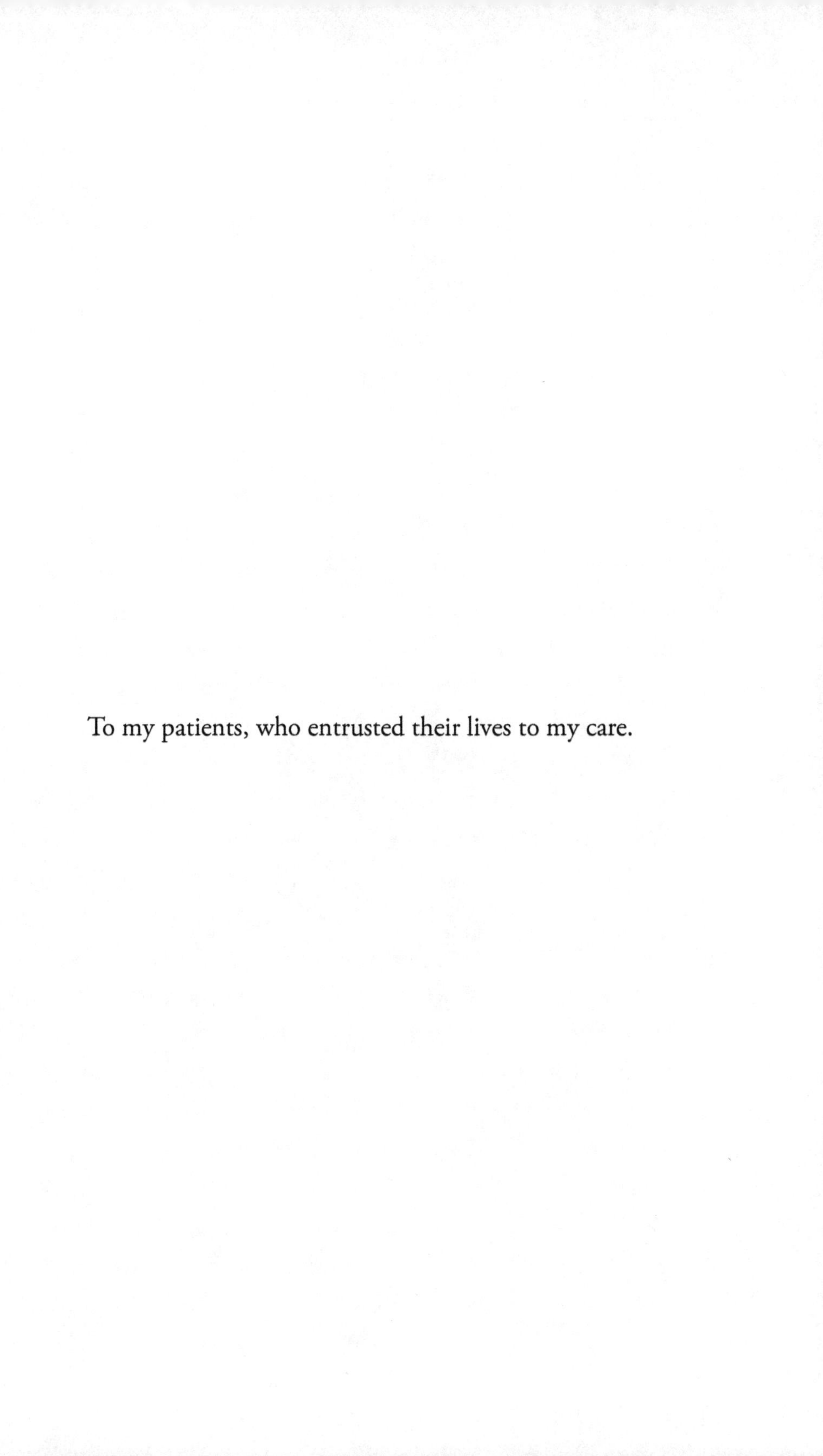

To my patients, who entrusted their lives to my care.

It was July 1986, and Billy Ocean's "There'll Be Sad Songs" was on top of the charts. *Ferris Bueller's Day Off* was showing at the movie theaters, and President Ronald Reagan presided over a relighting ceremony of a newly renovated Statue of Liberty. The Iran-Iraq War and the AIDS pandemic were in full swing, and I first stepped into a hospital as a member of the health-care team as a third-year medical student.

Compared to 2023, American medicine looked very different in 1986. Over these years, medicine has shifted from a system that rewards hospitals and doctors for what they do, too often without consideration as to whether it benefits patients or not, to a system that makes money by spending less, whether that harms patients or not. It's easy to see how neither system is desirable. You probably wouldn't take your car to the mechanic and say "Do whatever you think should be done" and hand over a blank check. However, you are probably no more likely to say, "Let's agree on what it's going to cost to work on my car, but I don't need to really know what you're going to do or whether it's going to fix the problem." As funny as it sounds, this is exactly where things have gone with American medicine. It's almost like we've all just said, "This is what we want to spend on medicine. Now you decide what that's going to get us, and we'll take it."

It's little wonder why we, as a society, have focused on controlling health-care costs. In the 1980s, US spending on healthcare was about 8.9% of gross domestic product; between 2010 and 2019, it averaged 17.4%. Health-care costs to individuals, out-of-pocket costs, and insurance premiums have doubled as well over this time frame after adjusting for inflation. Even more dramatically, I paid about $40,000 for medical school tuition whereas the median cost of medical school in 2019 to 2020 was $250,222 at public institutions and $330,180 at a private university. However, as we focus, almost exclusively, on controlling costs, we are heading down a dangerous and largely uncharted path.

A radical transformation of American healthcare has almost been completed. Accelerated by the COVID-19 pandemic, today, about 75% of doctors work for companies, typically hospitals or integrated health systems whereby hospitals and insurers are one. At the same time, hospitals are being paid not on the basis of the services they provide but on the labels they affix to patients. As reimbursement becomes fixed by a diagnosis label, profit is generated by spending less than the reimbursement for that label. When doctors are all employees of the system, patients have lost their most important advocate or, at the very least, that advocate is compromised by a duty to their employer.

It's true that when doctors and hospitals could profit by providing care, there was an incentive to provide unnecessary care and drive up costs. However, it's equally true that when these same providers can profit by spending less, there is an incentive to do less or use less-expensive and possibly less-effective treatments. We are facing a false choice between too much and not enough. If the incentives were better aligned so quality and outcomes were drivers of profit, patients would be much better served.

This book is about the false choices between having quality versus affordable healthcare. We can, like most other high-income countries, have both. It's about an untenable conflict of interest that exists when doctors are agents of a health-care system whose business model is counter to patient interests. It's about corruption at various levels within healthcare and about a gross misunderstanding on the part of government to fix the problem with solutions that are more likely to create new problems for patients.

Importantly, this book is not an exhaustive examination of the problems facing American medicine. Instead, it will examine one particularly troublesome problem that has been largely, if not totally, ignored by industry analysts and ethicists. It's a problem that is not currently on the radar of legislators who are almost always one step behind. And doctors, even the most ethical and well-meaning among us, are too often unaware or unable to appreciate the level of injustice that exists in the system that is emerging.

The year 1986 was also the year of the Space Shuttle Challenger disaster. The Challenger broke apart seventy-three seconds into its flight, killing all seven crew members aboard. Extensive investigation into the cause of the disaster revealed failure of the two redundant O-ring seals in the shuttle's right solid rocket booster. Record low temperatures at the time of the launch reduced the elasticity of the rubber O-rings, compromising them and leading to a breach of the joint shortly after liftoff. Pressurized gas from within the rocket booster leaked through the exposed joint and into the adjacent external fuel tank, leading to an explosion. The Rogers Commission was created to investigate the disaster, and it found that test data as early as 1977 had revealed a potentially catastrophic flaw in the O-rings. Neither NASA nor Morton Thiokol (the solid rocket booster manufacturer) addressed the issue. NASA managers also disregarded engineers' warnings about the dangers of launching in cold temperatures and did not report these technical concerns to their superiors.

We are facing a Challenger-style disaster in American healthcare. All the warning signs are there if we choose to examine them. Alternatively, we can continue to ignore the evidence and address the problem only after the disaster has occurred. There's big money in medicine, and no one wants to look too closely at how that money is being made. This book was written in the hope that we might still do the right thing. Before it's too late.

CHAPTER 1

Is She Really "My" Doctor?

Medicine cures diseases, but only doctors cure patients.

—Carl Jung

Over its history, even its recent history, American medicine has endured many crises. In 2007, Michael Moore took on the American health-care system with his documentary *Sicko*. The film makes the case for universal healthcare and focuses heavily on denial of care practices by insurance providers. However, even as the film was being released, the problem was shifting. Health insurance companies were already moving to a new tactic: limiting coverage to specific providers and inflating premiums even as they negotiated deep discounts with hospitals.

In his best-selling book *The Price We Pay: What Broke American Health Care—and How to Fix It*, Marty Makary, MD describes "the game" that hospitals and insurance companies play.[1] Hospitals inflate

---

[1] Marty Makary, MD, *The Price We Pay: What Broke American Health Care—and How to Fix It* (Bloomsbury Publishing, 2019).

bills more and more each year to generate more revenue because insurers only pay a fraction of the sticker price. Insurers, for their part, demand greater and greater discounts from hospitals to keep up and both pass on higher costs to the public in the form of co-payments and insurance premiums. Insurance companies, therefore, don't usually deny care. They cover patients within networks of hospitals and doctors where they have prenegotiated the costs. When patients are outside their insurance company networks or are uninsured completely, they find themselves at the mercy of hospitals who can essentially charge whatever they want. Yet, even as Dr. Makary's book was being published in 2019, the problem was already shifting again.

Although many of the problems identified by Makary and numerous others still very much exist today, new problems are emerging, and even some of the proposed solutions to older problems are creating these new problems. This book deals with one of the biggest and least acknowledged of these problems, and it affects all of us even when we are fully insured, in-network, and receiving care at hospitals with star ratings for fair pricing. Critically, this problem will not be solved by and will likely even worsen as a result of the proposed reforms, including value-based healthcare. Like a massive, multibillion-dollar Whack-a-Mole game, the problems in American healthcare are changing rapidly, and the media, congress, and even most experts are one step behind.

The problem I'm referring to is usually called a conflict of interest—a situation in which someone is involved in multiple interests, financial or otherwise, and serving one interest could involve working against another. Most often, this occurs because an individual's self-interest conflicts with an interest to serve someone else. Most consumers are aware of the potential for financial conflicts of interest inherent in all business transactions, and we are even on our guard for them most of time. For example, you want to have your kitchen remodeled, and you contact a general contractor who can manage the job. He comes to see you and meets you in your drabby kitchen, and you start talking about what changes you'd like to make. The conversation inevitably comes around to countertops and appliances. It's a kitchen remodel after all.

Now let's imagine that although you were thinking that new countertops and appliances would do the trick, the contractor recommends a complete redesign of the kitchen to make it more functional. Sure, it's going to be more expensive, but he's concerned about your happiness. Indeed, he might be concerned about your happiness, but if you are even a slightly savvy consumer, you are going to suspect that he might also be thinking about his bottom line. The redesign will make the project much bigger and more expensive. Does he have your interests at heart? Or does he see dollar signs? Actually, both may be true, and that's the inherent nature of the conflict. He's upselling you, sure, but you might very well be happier in the end if you take his advice.

Does this kind of conflict of interest take place in American fee-for-service medicine? Sure, it does. Do surgeons recommend surgery more often than nonsurgical doctors? Even if only by a small amount, there is no denying the potential for conflict of interest when a doctor, not just a surgeon but anyone performing a procedure, is recommending that procedure. Procedures pay better than advising a patient not to have a procedure. This is true 100% of the time. It's even true for just office visits. If a doctor recommends that she should see you back in three months to follow up on a problem she is treating you for, it is simultaneously true that this will serve you better, and it will bring in more money for the practice.

However, there are multiple ways of managing this conflict of interest, and because it is so familiar to us in the context of general commerce, society has developed various safeguards—whether or not those safeguards are usually effective. Indeed, the backbone of a free economy is competition, and one way this conflict of interest is managed is by having lots of options. If a second and a third contractor come to your house and provide you with different options, you are likely to find a solution that is tailored to your needs and not just the interests of the contractors. You are also likely to rate some of these contractors higher than others, and if you post reviews or just talk to your neighbors, the reputations of these contractors will be affected. Watchdog organizations like consumer reports also serve a role in helping to evaluate value in various products and services.

These same mechanisms can be helpful in healthcare as well, but there is a catch. Hospitals and insurance companies have shrouded their businesses in mystery and have greatly diminished the potential for competition. Your employer may not offer many choices for healthcare, and once you have an insurer, you may be very limited as to which hospital you can use. Reviews for health-care services can be helpful, but they are often driven by how friendly the office staff is and how easy it is to find parking. Nevertheless, you can read patient reviews for physicians you are considering and see if anyone is commenting on their business practices. You can also keep your eyes open.

I had a tooth broken while on vacation in Southern California, and a friend from the area recommended a dentist. The office was great. They got me in right away and treated me like an established patient. But I was blown away by the setup. It was one dentist in an office with a dozen rooms. He must have had a staff of twenty given all the people I saw. There was expensive-looking art hanging on the walls. When the dentist saw me, he immediately recommended an extraction of the remaining tooth and an implant. The tooth was fractured near the gumline, so this didn't seem unreasonable. Because I was only in town for a few days, though, he gave me a temporary crown and told me to follow up with my dentist back home for the extraction/implant procedure. However, when I saw my dentist back in Pittsburgh, who works out of an office in an old building with two examine rooms and a staff of two, he advised me to just start with a crown. I'm quite sure that the dentist in California would have told me that the crown is unlikely to work because the fracture was so close to the gumline, and it would be a waste of time and money to start with a crown when I would end up with an extraction/implant anyway. He may well have believed this and may have trained in dentistry in a setting where the community standard was for more aggressive use of implants compared to where my dentist trained. However, there is no denying that the extraction/implant route would be far more lucrative for the dentist. This all happened to me more than ten years ago. I still have that crown in my mouth today.

This example with my own dental woes illustrates the difficulty in judging the motivations of health-care providers on a case-by-case basis. As a result, there are other safeguards. Consumer watchdog organizations are active in the health-care space, but their effectiveness is limited. *U. S. News & World Report* has been ranking US hospitals since 1990. However, until rather recently, their methodology was purely subjective. Basically, it's a survey of doctors as to which hospitals they think are best. Given that most doctors surveyed are employed by hospitals, it's a rather strange way of determining what hospitals are "best." Although *U. S. News & World Report* has begun to incorporate objective criteria in its rankings, it's still a very flawed system.

Top Doctors is actually worse. Their system involves nominating doctors who then accept the nomination by filling out a profile. When I was nominated, the profile was pretty basic—education, practice location, board certification, the sort of information anyone can provide. There were no objective criteria for differentiating me as a "top" doctor as opposed to all the other physicians in the area. As soon as I became a "top doctor," I started receiving emails inviting me to select the kind of plaque that I wanted to buy, starting at the basic one-hundred-dollar version to a variety of nicer and more expensive ones. It became rather obvious that the purpose of the program was to sell advertising to doctors and perhaps to pander to their vanity. After a couple of years of ignoring the plaque offers, I dropped off the list. *Who's Who in America* works pretty much the same way. The business model is about selling a directory, not about informing the public in any meaningful way.

A more effective safeguard against medical profiteering, therefore, is the profession itself. Published standards, usually based on scientific evidence, drive practice patterns in most communities. This is only partially effective, however, because it relies on self-policing to follow the standards, and just like the contractor who wants to upsell you on your kitchen, a physician may still find a way to recommend a procedure against published standards. Thus, the most important safeguard against this form of conflict of interest, whether it's in home remolding or healthcare, is an informed consumer. The fact that most of us don't pay for medical care directly but do so indirectly through medical insurance can provide an additional layer of safeguard. Indeed "pre-authorization" policies for various medical procedures are often justified on the basis that they can reduce unnecessary spending. Whether this is true or not is unclear, but they do provide additional scrutiny over physician recommendations. We, as consumers, may rely on this too much, however. Chances are if a doctor recommends something to us and our insurance provider is willing to pay for it, we might not think twice about it. Indeed, when patients are surveyed about their attitudes toward their physicians, only a small minority report being concerned about financial motives.

Importantly, though, this more overt conflict of interest, where the physician or hospital is effectively upselling services, is not the only type of conflict of interest that exists and may not even be the most dangerous. Unfortunately, there's a really good chance (and this chance has been increasing rapidly in the last decade) that your doctor has a different type of conflict of interest. This type of conflict of interest is not upselling. It's just the opposite, and it's not being discussed by lawmakers, professional societies, or even ethicists to any degree. It's become ingrained in the fabric of American medicine from the humblest of clinics all the way to the most prestigious hospitals. In fact, it's especially insidious at top hospitals and among the "top doctors in America." The conflict does not directly involve doctors' own financial interests though there are very strong indirect links. Instead, the conflict is between your interests as a patient and the interests of your doctor's employer. That's right. In America, the majority of doctors no longer own their practices, and even those who do often enter into financial arrangements that create a very real and largely undisclosed conflict of interest.

Lawmakers and professional watchdog organizations primarily concern themselves with policing physician relationships with outside entities, particularly drug and device manufacturers. While these relationships can and sometimes do pose real threats to the best interests of patients—discussed further in chapter 5—they pale in comparison, both in scope and potential for harm, to the systemic conflicts of interest built into modern American medicine.

In this book, I will explore how doctors have become accomplices, usually unwitting, in what has become a multibillion-dollar system to defraud patients and taxpayers of health-care dollars. I will consider the fundamental flaws and misinformation, which have permitted this system to develop and grow, and the lies that perpetuate it. Finally, I will lay out a series of much-needed reforms for the system as a whole and specific steps patients and doctors can take to avoid as much as possible employer-based financial conflicts of interest. I mention doctors in my prescription for fixing this aspect of American medicine because, as I will examine in depth in later chapters, the vast majority of us physicians don't actually want to work in the system that has evolved and instead want to work on behalf of patients and to have their best interests at heart. I will also try to explain why the current system is as bad for doctors as it is for patients and how both have enjoyed certain benefits from this system that have served to obscure the very real harm it has done.

Thankfully, reforming the system need not sacrifice the benefits that a corporate health-care delivery approach has brought to American medicine—such as efficiency, integration, and possibly improved safety. However, reform must acknowledge the harm this system has brought forth and how a system that is primarily concerned with profit, as corporations are, will only deliver the best care to patients if the profit incentives are intimately aligned with patient's interests, and currently, they are not. In the process, I will compare and contrast various institutions and models of care both within the United States and abroad. These comparisons will help illustrate how differences in priorities and incentives can influence how care is provided and also illustrate how and why no system is perfect. However, in many ways, healthcare in the United States is inferior to other systems in high-income countries. That's right. We rank dead last in comparison to most systems in countries with similar means—all the while we rank first in the cost of healthcare. Of course, if you are selling healthcare, this is a pretty good deal. If you are consumer, though, you will no doubt wonder how this has happened and what can be done to fix it.

In reality, though, our system functions perfectly as designed, well, not as designed perhaps, but as it has evolved to be. Our system maximizes profits for large corporations that were gradually and are now rapidly controlling health-care delivery in the United States and changing the culture one hospital and one physician practice at a time. By buying physician practices, essentially buying the doctor's patients, the large corporate entity makes the physician an employee. Through a system of control and subtle and not-so-subtle coercion, the corporation can dictate which treatments are offered and which ones are not. Part of the process is to use the tools of science to make these decisions seem entirely appropriate and not in the service of the institution's bottom line. Sometimes these directives are very appropriate and serve to improve patient outcomes. Just as often, though, treatment decisions are made to maximize profit, usually by reducing costs, while maintaining revenue and not "greatly lowering" quality.

As I will discuss later on, a system known as evidence-based medicine, while serving to make care more scientific, has been corrupted in many instances to make care more economical for providers and payors. Often, researchers express benefit or lack of benefit from a certain therapy in terms of the number needed to treat (NNT) to achieve a desired outcome. Drugs and devices are approved by regulatory bodies, like the US Food and Drug Administration, based on their indications for use. If a drug is intended to prevent a potentially fatal illness like a myocardial infarction, a heart attack, then the NNT would be calculated on the number of patients who would need to be treated to prevent one myocardial infarction. Blood thinners like heparin can be used in patients with unstable angina (heart pain at rest), and the NNT to prevent one myocardial infarction is about thirty-three. The larger this number is, the smaller the effect of the intervention because more people need to be treated to achieve one success. If the intervention causes serious adverse effects, researchers may also calculate the NNH (number needed to harm). For heparin, bleeding occurs in about one in seventeen patients (NNH = 17). These are mainly minor, non-life-threatening bleeding events, however, so it's a judgment call as to whether an NNT for myocardial infarction of thirty-three is beneficial when the NNH for bleeding is seventeen. If you consider bleeding of this sort to be half as serious as a heart attack, then you would conclude that the benefit (one in thirty-three) and the risk (one in seventeen times two or one in thirty-four) are nearly identical. Thus, this therapy should not be used. Indeed, other outcomes like survival are not improved with heparin either; therefore, heparin is not usually recommended for this indication.

In general, if the NNT and a similarly significant NNH are close to each (or if the risks are actually greater than the benefit), the intervention will not be recommended. More often, though, NNT is far lower (meaning greater benefit because fewer patients are required to have a positive outcome) than NNH. However, if the intervention is expensive, a health-care economist, using very strict rules of analysis, might argue that an intervention is not "cost-effective" or, simply put, is not worth the cost. For example, if a therapy with an NNT of one hundred were to cost ten thousand dollars per patient, the cost of achieving one desired outcome would be one hundred times ten thousand or one million dollars. I'll explain the details of this analysis later, but its use is not limited to healthcare. The same rules have been used to determine the cost-effectiveness of airbags, for example, and this analysis has not only been used to justify their use but even to make them mandatory on new cars. From a societal perspective, there is a great need to put healthcare in a cost-effectiveness framework. When interventions are very expensive or even when they are only moderately expensive but are very common such that the total costs become significant, society has the right to ask, "Is this the best way to use limited resources?" Unfortunately, very few physicians and almost no hospital administrators are health-care economists. Instead, these individuals may fall into the trap of "healthcare accounting." Unlike economics, accounting only measures costs, which are easy to quantify, without careful consideration of value.

Take for example a new medication for putting patients to sleep for surgery (we'll call it Gut-easy) that does exactly what the old medication does (let's call it RoughStuff). In this example, let's say that Gut-easy, the new medication, is no more effective for anesthesia than RoughStuff. As such, we don't need to worry about how to factor in effectiveness—the NNT is the same for both drugs. However, let's also say that Gut-easy has significantly fewer adverse effects. For example, let's say that this medication causes nausea in only 1% of patients whereas the old medication, RoughStuff, causes this effect in 30%—hence the name. From a patient perspective, there is great value in not being nauseous. However, from a strict accounting perspective, there is only the cost of Gut-easy versus the cost of RoughStuff. Nausea does not have a cost that can be measured. If, on the other hand, the Gut-easy, with its better tolerability, resulted in a shorter hospital stay, the health-care accountant could discount the total costs of care including the more expensive drug compared to the older drug. In such cases, there is a "win-win," such that the patient benefits from less nausea, and in a system where revenue is fixed by diagnosis rather than utilization, a shorter hospital stay saves money for the hospital.

Unfortunately, not all interventions can be shown to be cost-saving or even cost-neutral; thus, adoption of new therapy relies on other factors. Traditionally, a major factor driving adoption was advocacy by physicians. As patient advocates, doctors could push for therapies that were in patients' best interests even if they were not in line with hospitals' financial interests. This was always a delicate balance, of course. If a new drug was requested by a doctor, she or he would be expected to explain why it should be available to patients. If the drug was only slightly more expensive, the justification might be trivial (e.g., it requires dosing once a day as opposed to twice a day). If the new drug was more expensive, a more persuasive rationale might be needed. However, hospitals would generally take heed of physician recommendations for two important reasons: First, hospital administrators, while possibly physicians themselves, largely left the practice of medicine to doctors. Second, a physician in private practice could choose which hospital to admit her or his patients to, thus having some leverage with individual hospitals.

However, gradually, the balance of power has shifted. Hospital administrators are now rarely physicians themselves, and although they still rely on doctors to make medical decisions, they have placed some of the decision-making power in the hands of small groups of doctors rather than leaving care decisions to individual physicians. One example of this is Pharmacy and Therapeutics (P&T) committees. P&T committees are generally composed of pharmacists and physicians, and together they determine hospital formularies. Formularies are essentially the menu of drugs and devices that are stocked by the hospital. By limiting hospital formularies, hospitals can control costs in two ways: First, because the purchase of some drugs can be bundled together, a hospital can get discounts when it limits the number of different drugs it needs to buy. The second way formularies can control costs is by not including expensive drugs. If a drug is not on the formulary, it is essentially not available to be ordered by doctors.

On the face of it, it may not seem that putting decision-making power in the hands of small groups of doctors is that different from leaving the decisions to each doctor. However, because the hospital determines who sits on the P&T committee, it can essentially "pack the court" to ensure that the decisions are favorable to the hospital's bottom line. The aggressiveness by which this occurs can be startling. Most hospitals exclude at least some drugs from their formularies altogether, and for other drugs, they may have strict processes that have to be followed for these drugs to be used. For example, the hospital may use gatekeepers to limit the use of some drugs. These gatekeepers may be specialists in certain areas of medicine, and it's often easy for hospitals to justify restricting certain medications for safety reasons. However, this method can also be used to reduce costs to the system.

But how are doctors coerced into making these decisions that are possibly bad for patients just to save a few dollars for hospitals? The answer to this question is complex, and I will explore it in detail in chapter 6. However, the basic problem can be illustrated using a simple example:

Dr. Smith and Dr. Jones are both emergency medicine physicians who both practice in a similar way. Both doctors are asked to reduce their prescribing of a specific medicine and, when it's "medically appropriate," to use a less-expensive alternative. The hospital may not try to tell the doctors when it's medically appropriate—it may not need to.

Dr. Smith decides that 90% of her patients should continue to receive the more expensive drug, conceding that 10% are appropriate to receive a less-expensive alternative. However, Dr. Jones believes that, virtually, none of her patients require the more expensive drug she has been using and converts 99% to the lower-cost drug. Other doctors working at this hospital have a range of opinions and compliance with the hospital's request, and they fall in line somewhere between Dr. Smith and Dr. Jones.

In her annual review, Dr. Jones is praised for her efforts to control costs in the hospital while Dr. Smith is told that her use of an expensive drug is far in excess of the average of her peers. She is then asked to reevaluate her prescribing practices. Dr. Smith may take the hint and reduce her use of the expensive drug to at least come "in line" with her peers, but she may decide that she is unwilling to compromise her professional judgment. The hospital may then promote Dr. Jones and not Dr. Smith or give Dr. Jones a better schedule or other benefits that it denies Dr. Smith. The reasons cited for these decisions may actually include the fact that Dr. Jones is cost-conscious, and Dr. Smith is not. Alternatively, the hospital may communicate in more subtle language. Dr. Jones's evaluations may indicate that she is a "team player" or "always appreciates the big picture." Dr. Smith's evaluations may say the opposite.

Of course, the hospital or university doesn't have to even mention this issue when it's evaluating doctors for raises, promotions, or other considerations, including retention, yet the issue may still be influencing important decisions that impact the doctor's career. The evaluation process for professionals is often extremely subjective, and Dr. Smith's supervisor may not even intentionally factor in issues of cost-consciousness in his or her evaluation of Dr. Smith's performance. Even more importantly, the supervisor, let's call her Dr. Miller, is likely to have an indirect (or even a direct) financial interest in the outcome of efforts to control costs in the emergency department in which Dr. Jones and Dr. Smith work. Dr. Miller may have received a directive to reduce the use of a specific drug or, more commonly, Dr. Miller may have been told to reduce the costs in her department by a certain percentage. Dr. Miller may have looked at drug costs as a good target to reduce "waste" and may have chosen a couple of expensive medications to reduce. Estimation of Dr. Miller's performance as the director of the emergency department may be strongly coupled to her ability to control costs. She may be removed as the director if she's unable to perform well in this capacity. Of course, she will be well-aware of this, and although she may not speak of it directly to the doctors reporting to her, the fact always underpins interactions between them. If Dr. Smith doesn't "come in line," her actions will likely jeopardize Dr. Miller's ability to achieve the cost reductions she is being asked to make. Failure to make these targets may get Dr. Miller fired. Obviously, any evaluation of Dr. Smith's performance by Dr. Miller is going to be colored by this fact. Indeed, Dr. Miller has a financial conflict of interest when making assessments as to Dr. Smith's performance, which will impact her likelihood of being promoted, receiving raises, or even being retained on staff.

The financial conflicts of interest among hospital administrators, whether they are doctors or not, may be even more direct. In the above example, Dr. Miller may receive a bonus based on her ability to make the cost-reduction targets or lose money if she does not. That's right. Dr. Miller might actually have her pay cut if she doesn't meet the target. Financial incentives may also reach right down to the frontline doctors, and they may be quite nasty. For example, the emergency-department doctors might all have a portion of their salary "at risk." They may all lose this money if certain targets are not met. These might include important patient-centered outcomes like satisfaction and safety, but they might also include things that directly influence the hospital's bottom line like how many patients a doctor sees in a shift. They may also cover the use of certain medications or procedures. If Dr. Smith causes the group to miss its target, the whole staff may be financially impacted. Obviously, this is going to make Dr. Smith's life rather miserable.

Many doctors in the US have performance-based pay, and this represents yet another conflict of interest. In general, doctors make more money if they bill more. This produces a financial incentive for a doctor to perform a surgical or complex medical procedure because the doctor earns more money when he or she does the procedure. This is the type of conflict of interest discussed above, and it has been around since ancient times. To a certain degree, this kind of conflict of interest is inevitable in a fee-for-service environment. For this reason, there are multiple laws, regulations, and practices (e.g., second opinions) that help manage this type of conflict, and as discussed above, the public is at least aware of it. However, most patients would be stunned to learn that their doctor or his boss might get a bonus if they prescribe a cheaper medication. In essence, because the total payment for a hospitalization is based on the diagnosis, hospitals get a fixed price for caring for you. If they can cut corners and reduce the cost, they can turn a profit on the whole transaction. Now if they were to use that money to lower the price, which, in turn, lowered your insurance premium or your out-of-pocket expenses, you might even agree to this. There are some systems in which this happens to a degree. You might even be agreeable if the hospital were to plough the profits back into improving patient care. However, more often than not, the health system is just pocketing this profit and often paying exorbitant bonuses to their executives.

According to a report in Becker's Hospital Review,[2] in 2020, the highest-paid health-care executive was listed as Amir Rubin from 1Life Healthcare, doing business as One Medical. He reportedly earned $199,053,051 in just that year. However, the company told Becker's that Mr. Rubin's salary was 1.6 million in 2020, and the rest of the reported earnings was through a "performance-based equity grant." Of course, we don't know the structure of this incentive, but since hospital revenues for each patient are more or less fixed, profits are largely a function of reducing costs. Thus, it's fair to assume that Mr. Rubin's bonuses were funded by cost savings to the system. So the next time you or someone close to you receives an off-brand medication or medical device including bandages, catheters, etc., you can be confident that someone is getting what amounts to a kickback on the cost savings. How does that make you feel?

At this point, you may be wondering how this could happen, how it could be legal, and why the US government isn't doing anything about it. Let's start with the last part: Why isn't the government addressing this?

Although there may be several potential explanations including inefficiency of government agencies, political concerns, lobbying, and general governmental ineffectiveness, an important consideration is that the government is the single largest payor of healthcare.

---

[2] https://www.beckershospitalreview.com/rankings-and-ratings/the-7-highest-paid-health-system-ceos.html.

As such, the government has its own conflict of interest. Although the cost savings that we are discussing do not get funneled back to the payors since the payments are fixed by the diagnosis, there is a pervasive assumption that lowering costs will permit payors, including the federal government, to hold down cost increases from year to year. Although the US spends considerably more for healthcare as a percentage of gross domestic product (about 17%) than other countries (on average, European countries spend less than 9%), this has been relatively stable for the last few years up until the start of the COVID-19 pandemic unlike the massive increases seen previously. For example, in 2000, national healthcare expenditures in the US were about 12.5% of gross domestic product (GDP) and rose to just under 16.3% in 2009. Whereas in the next nine years, this proportion only increased to 16.9%. Importantly, unlike hospital systems and private payors, the federal government doesn't use cost savings in the health-care budget to pay a small number of people exorbitant sums. In this regard, if the feds can hold down health-care costs, we may all benefit since we are the ones ultimately footing the bill.

Unfortunately, while the US government and other payors are closely watching health-care spending, little scrutiny is placed on hospital profits, and this includes revenue for nonprofit and for-profit institutions. According to the US Census Bureau, total revenue for hospitals has been growing sharply for many years.[3] Industry-wide, total revenues for the first quarter of 2005 were $152 billion, increasing to $196 billion by the last quarter of 2009. By the end of 2019, revenues had reached over $300 billion a quarter. Data on hospital spending are less easy to find; therefore, calculating hospital profits

---

[3] https://fred.stlouisfed.org/series/REV622ALLEST144QSA.

can be difficult. However, by far, the largest cost that hospitals have is labor. Over the same decade that hospital revenues increased by more than 50%, average physician salaries increased by only 21%, and nursing pay increased by less than 15%. Conversely, executive salaries soared so much that by 2020, total compensation for health-system CEOs routinely exceeded ten million dollars per year. While hospitals spend money on many other things, these numbers make it apparent that going into the COVID-19 pandemic, hospital balance sheets were, on average, in pretty good shape.

This conclusion is also supported by National Health Expenditure (NHE) data. According to an analysis by the Peterson Center on Healthcare, a nonprofit health-care watchdog, hospital spending in the 1970s grew at a staggering 14% per year, outpacing GDP by 5%. This growth eased somewhat in the 1980s but was still nearly 10% per year. However, over the last decade, the annual increase in hospital spending has been under 5%.[4] Thus, even with exorbitant executive salaries, hospital revenues and spending have been closely matched for the last several years.

Of course, this will come as no surprise to anyone with an Internet connection or access to newspapers or television. The news media has run multiple stories on record profits of various hospital systems over the last several years. However, for those working within these organizations, a very different picture is painted. Whether the story is that "the media doesn't see the whole picture" or that "yes, profits are up this quarter, but it's only because of certain factors that are nonrecurring" or any number of other explanations, everyone

---

[4]   https://www.healthsystemtracker.org/chart-collection/u-s-spending-healthcare-changed-time/.

working in healthcare is constantly reminded that their hospital or system is just one or two bad quarters away from disaster. After all, in the long run, most hospitals lose money, don't they? This idea is the essence of "the *big lie* in healthcare"; essentially, that hospitals are on the brink of insolvency and, therefore, need to charge more and pay less in workforce salaries. It's actually quite astonishing how hospital administrators are able to spin their finances to justify austerity measures while simultaneously paying themselves bonuses. Their ability to do this is helped in no small measure by the complexity and opaqueness of hospital billing and reimbursement.

The *big lie* in healthcare is quite pervasive and explains how hospitals can convince doctors and, to a lesser extent, pharmacists, nurses, and all other hospital professionals that they have to be very careful not to spend more on a patient than they can be reimbursed. Of course, none of these frontline workers knows what the reimbursement is, so the result is that whenever someone in administration asks that something not be used, providers simply agree. Only when it is very clear that withholding something would directly and adversely impact the patient does anyone question the directive. Even then, it may be difficult to determine the implications because the directive is usually not to withhold a therapy but instead to use a cheaper alternative. Even when the cheaper alternative is known to be less effective, clinicians may be willing to use it on the grounds that the more expensive therapy isn't *so much* better that it justifies bankrupting the hospital. The fact that many physicians are employed by said hospital makes the connection between hospital economics and physician pay anything but abstract. In chapter 4, I will examine the foundations of the *big lie* in healthcare and how hospital executives manage to use this well-established myth to coerce physicians and other providers to make costs a primary consideration in clinical decision-making.

In the outpatient world, costs might be discussed with patients in the context of their insurance coverage. Patients might ask, "Will my prescription drug benefit cover the cost of this new medication?" or "What will my out-of-pocket expense be for this treatment?" However, in the hospital, patients are never consulted regarding costs; therefore, any cost-consciousness on the part of providers is strictly for the benefit of hospitals, not patients. Cost containment is, of course, not inherently evil, but there is certainly something sinister about not involving patients in decisions that can affect their health and pocketing the cost savings.

Throughout this book, I will examine how the current practice of medicine has become corrupted by corporate executives and hospital administrators and how the system harms patients and places physicians in an untenable conflict of interest. I will also provide a basic road map to reform the system and consider specific steps patients and doctors can take to avoid as much as possible employer-based financial conflicts of interest. Healthcare in America didn't used to be like this, and it doesn't have to stay this way.

CHAPTER 2

The Problem Is the Business Model

*We'll go down in history as the first society that wouldn't
save itself because it wasn't cost-effective.*

—Kurt Vonnegut

A fundamental problem that our current health-care system faces is that hospitals make money based on a business model that is counter to their customers' interests. It impacts every aspect of how hospitals operate. Insurance providers can make money by charging premiums and reducing claims either through keeping their clients healthy (good) or denying services (bad). Hospitals, by contrast, are more constrained. They cannot make money by keeping patients healthy. In fact, they lose money when patients require less care. Hospitals make money either by charging more or spending less—often both at the same time. Hospitals charge more by maximizing the codes used to bill insurance, including Medicare. This is highly technical and has prompted hospitals to hire entire departments to maximize coding (which further increases their costs). It's also risky for the hospital because if they are too aggressive with Medicare, they can be charged with fraud. They are much less constrained when it comes to private insurance, but they have prenegotiated fees in the form of managed care. They can and do charge much higher rates to uninsured patients (including those with insurance they do not accept), but these patients are usually the minority, and many uninsured or underinsured simply can't pay anyway. Still, an estimated one in five households have unpaid medical bills totaling eighty-eight billion dollars as of June 2021, according to a report by the Consumer Financial Protection Bureau. It's unknown how many hospitals turn these unpaid bills over to collection agencies, but many do, and some hospitals have even gone to courts to garnish wages.

And then there is so-called Medicare Advantage, the private-sector alternative to original Medicare. Today, nearly half of all Medicare beneficiaries are enrolled in Medicare Advantage. The program is controversial and politically charged. While most of its subscribers like the extra benefits many plans provide, the program costs the federal government and, hence, taxpayers significantly more than the original public program. Furthermore, while seniors are enticed into these plans with shockingly low premiums, some even zero dollars per month, when they get sick, Medicare Advantage participants may find that their overall costs skyrocket due to co-payments and out-of-pocket expenses. This has led some critics to charge that the only advantage of the program seems to be to the private insurers.

Indeed, major insurers have made no secret about how lucrative the program can be. Humana, one of the nation's largest health insurers recently said it would leave the commercial insurance market and focus on government-funded programs, like its booming Medicare Advantage plans. And it's not hard to see why these plans can be so lucrative. First, private insurers receive a fixed amount each month from Medicare for each patient they cover. However, these companies can still turn around and charge policyholders various co-payments and out-of-pocket costs and are able to establish their own rules for service, such as the need for referrals or provider networks for both nonurgent care and emergency services. While Medicare Advantage plans must "accept" any Medicare-eligible participant, some discourage people at greatest need, those with more health issues, by the way they structure their co-payments and deductibles. Many enrollees have been hit with unexpected costs and denial of benefits for various types of care deemed not medically necessary. In essence, it's a perfect arrangement if you are an insurance company. Not so much if you are a sick patient or taxpayer.

It is important to realize that hospitals are paid largely on the basis of the diagnostic category (or group) a patient can be placed in and not based on the care the patient receives. The category is influenced by whether certain procedures are performed (most surgeries, for instance), but the amount a hospital is paid for a given case may bear little resemblance to the number of services provided. Consider the following example:

David Johnson is a sixty-eight-year-old smoker who develops severe pneumonia and is hospitalized. Given the severity of his pneumonia and his underlying lung disease from smoking, he requires intubation (insertion of a breathing tube) and mechanical ventilation. For this, he is admitted to the intensive care unit. After two days, his condition is improved, and his doctors are attempting to see if he can be taken off the ventilator and breathe on his own. He's making progress, but it's still not clear if he's ready. On one hand, the doctor can choose to remove the tube and see how David does. This puts him at a slightly increased risk because the tube may have to be reinserted, and he may become unstable during this period. On the other hand, the longer he's on the ventilator, the more sedation he will require, and the weaker his body will get.

There are reasonable medical arguments both for removing the tube now or waiting another day and reevaluating. However, there's also an economic argument. Right now, the hospital can bill for a "respiratory system diagnosis with mechanical ventilation" (DRG 208). This pays about twenty-two thousand dollars. Mr. Johnson has a severe infection with respiratory failure, so he also meets the criteria for ICD-10-CM R65.21: "severe sepsis." This pays about ten thousand dollars more. If he can be removed from the ventilator, he will be able to leave the ICU and markedly reduce the cost to the hospital for his care.

ICUs are expensive with high nurse-to-patient ratios and lots of ancillary services, including respiratory therapists, more intensive pharmacist staffing, etc. So if the patient spends another day in the ICU, it might cost the hospital an extra two thousand dollars, but the payment to the hospital will still be the same. However, if the patient stays on the ventilator for two more days (more than ninety-six hours total), the hospital can bill DRG 207, "respiratory system diagnosis with mechanical ventilation >96 hours," which pays more than twice as much.

It's easy to see how the hospital would be incentivized to make sure patients are removed from the ventilator at ninety-seven hours rather than ninety-five. In truth, as an ICU doctor, I have never been asked to keep a patient on the ventilator to meet this criterion. In fact, all the hospitals I've worked in actually try to shorten the duration of mechanical ventilation. Still, a potential for conflict of interest exists.

A more common and controversial issue concerns the use of tracheostomy in patients like Mr. Johnson. A tracheostomy is a minor surgical procedure in which a smaller tube is inserted directly into the trachea through a small incision at the base of the neck. When this is done, the patient can breathe through this tube and have the larger tube removed from the throat. Most patients find this much more comfortable, and patients can be removed and reattached to the ventilator without removing the tube, which improves the safety of attempts to breathe without the ventilator. Many hospitals and professional societies have advocated for earlier use of tracheostomy to reap these benefits. However, the use of tracheostomy also allows the hospital to bill DRG 004, "tracheostomy with mechanical ventilation >96 hours," which pays more than twice DRG 207. Again, I personally have never been asked to perform a tracheostomy on a patient to improve the hospital's reimbursement nor have I been aware of anyone else encountering this request. However, I have worked at multiple hospitals with protocols in place to encourage early use of tracheostomy citing patient-centered benefits. While I'm prepared to believe that the primary motivation for these protocols is the benefit to the patient, it's doubtful that hospitals are unaware of the financial benefits to the organization.

When hospitals can influence clinical practice and at the same time influence the amount of payment they can receive, a serious potential for abuse exists. There will always be some situations where a clinical argument can be made to do or not do something. If financial influence can impact this decision, even indirectly, there is a conflict of interest. As hospitals employ more and more clinicians, they have greater and greater control over just these clinical decisions, and the potential for abuse rises dramatically. Making physicians and physician extenders independent of hospitals and precluding hospitals from influencing clinical decision-making is needed to help manage this risk.

Thus, there are numerous ways that hospitals can manipulate charges under a diagnosis-related group (DRG) system that can be hard to disentangle from appropriate charges for appropriate and necessary care. Another problem exists when a patient is uninsured or has insurance but is receiving care in a situation where they are not covered, a condition referred to as out of network. In such situations, hospitals are not obliged to follow any pricing guidelines. They can essentially charge whatever they want. While inflated pricing (which some would rightly call price gouging) is a huge problem for patients caught in these situations, it's already a target of reform. At the time of writing this, Congress recently enacted legislation to help address one major aspect of the problem so-called "surprise" bills. Effective January 1, 2022, the No Surprises Act (NSA) protects consumers from surprise billing if they have a group health plan or group or individual health insurance coverage. The act specifically bans surprise bills for emergency services from an out-of-network provider or facility unless patients agree to such costs up front. We'll examine this legislation in detail later, but it's important to note that most surprise, out-of-network emergency charges are from doctors and other out-of-network professionals including air ambulance services rather than from the hospital or emergency facilities themselves. Thus, while surprise bills are a major problem (one study found that 18% of emergency-department visits resulted in at least one out-of-network charge), they pale in comparison to the problems discussed here because employer-based conflicts of interest have the potential to affect 100% of visits.

No doubt, some hospitals do make profits on out-of-network charges. However, from a hospital perspective, a better approach is to cut costs by reducing the use of expensive drugs and equipment by maximizing patient-to-provider ratios and reducing payroll. When hospitals hold their charges steady, they make their profits by reducing their costs. Government agencies and the press often refer to these cost-cutting measures as reducing waste. Indeed, there has been and continues to be wasteful spending in healthcare. Waste in this context can be defined as providing services that are "low value," meaning that cost-to-benefit ratio is high. The problem here is that while the costs can easily be calculated, there is plenty of subjectivity in determining benefit. Being in the hospital is generally an unpleasant experience for most people even under the best of circumstances. There is pain and discomfort, loss of autonomy, sleep disruption, food that we may not enjoy, and a host of other inconveniences that we are expected to endure.

A commonly used, low-cost pain relief medicine is acetaminophen, trade name Tylenol. If you have ever taken acetaminophen to treat acute pain like from an orthopedic injury such as a sprained ankle or a fractured bone, you may be surprised at how well it works. However, when we are sick in the hospital, we may not be able to take oral medication. The alternatives include other drugs, all of which have more side effects; acetaminophen suppository, which most find unpleasant; or a relatively new formulation of acetaminophen that can be given intravenously. Interestingly, because intravenous acetaminophen doesn't need to be absorbed from either end of our gastrointestinal tract, the relief is nearly instantaneous. Some patients find intravenous acetaminophen even more effective than narcotics, and obviously, it's much, much safer. What would you pay for this therapy if you were having acute pain and you could not take a pill? Unfortunately, you are not likely to be asked. Instead, someone or, more likely, a committee at the hospital will decide whether the benefits of this drug are worth the costs. Because it's new, this form of acetaminophen is expensive. Let's say it costs about seventy dollars more per dose. Your risk of death or disability from receiving an acetaminophen suppository as opposed to an injection is essentially zero, so many hospitals will simply decide that your discomfort isn't worth the seventy dollars. In truth, you might even agree. On the other hand, if you participate in this "waste" elimination process, shouldn't you expect to receive a discount on your health insurance premium? After all, you paid for the insurance; the hospital is paid the same whether they give you one therapy or the other. Why should the hospital get to make more profit at your expense?

Furthermore, some of the care that we are provided can have long-lasting effects on our health and even on our survival. Let's say you can't have a suppository either. What then? There are, of course, other drugs to treat pain. However, these drugs all have side effects, and usually, the side effects are more pronounced or more consequential the sicker we are. As a doctor caring for patients in an intensive care unit, I have actually been prohibited from prescribing intravenous acetaminophen to patients on the grounds that it's too expensive. In each of these cases, it was possible to provide the acetaminophen by another route, either by suppository or into the stomach by way of a tube. However, had I instead prescribed an alternative agent, there is a small but measurable risk of causing real harm. If I look at this risk as a patient, I might decide that seventy dollars is worth spending to mitigate even a small risk. If I look at this as a hospital, however, I may instead decide that if the risk was, say, one in one thousand, seventy thousand dollars would be spent to avoid just one serious adverse event, such as kidney failure or major bleeding. It's possible that the hospital might conclude that it's not worth it. But is this really waste?

Hospitals also adjust staffing to save money. If a hospital can pull one nurse out of a unit, it can save the costs of salary and benefits for that nurse. When I completed my intensive care training in the 1990s, ICUs were staffed so there was either one or two patients for each nurse depending on how sick the patients were. Sicker patients got their own nurse while less-sick patients shared a nurse with another patient. Furthermore, a senior-level nurse was often assigned to the unit as a resource to the whole unit so if an extra set of hands was needed, they were readily available and didn't need to come from another bedside. Over the intervening years, this "extra nurse" was assigned less frequently and then not at all. Staffing has moved from mainly 1:1 with an occasional 1:2 to now where it is almost all 1:2 with an occasional 1:3!

Another target for "waste reduction" is new technology. Again, when I finished my ICU training, the purchase of new technology was largely, if not exclusively, driven by clinician request. If I wanted a new tool for my patients, I was usually not asked why, and it was usually provided. There was a sense, even then, that the new technology should be necessary, and if it ended up gathering dust in the corner, someone would ask about it. But this was the extent of the process. Today, there are "value assessment teams" or VATs that evaluate all new technology requests. The VAT works to ensure that purchasing of new equipment brings value to the system. Notice the wording here. Value "to the system." Typical VATs do not have a mandate to bring value to patients.

Not only do all these practices fail to benefit patients but they may also actually work against their interests. Innovation is expensive, especially in drugs and medical devices. By disincentivizing hospitals to adopt new technology, patients do not get access to the latest advances in medicine or get them as quickly as they should, and usually, patients don't even know it. Furthermore, maximizing patient-to-provider ratios and reducing staff put the burden on patients who must contend with long wait times, crowded conditions, and often providers who are rushed, stressed, and unhappy. Almost nothing in the business model aligns with patient satisfaction, so this aspect is usually only an afterthought or focused on specific patient types where the hospital wishes to grow its business. Furthermore, patient satisfaction is usually a function of service, not outcomes. Medicine is complex, and most patients can't judge how well they are cared for, only *how* they are cared for. A hospital that consistently performs well in terms of clinical outcomes will still suffer in the public eye if the food in the cafeteria is bad or parking is unavailable. For this reason, hospitals are just as likely to invest in modernizing their physical plant than they are in hiring and retaining the most talented clinicians.

It should be said that containing costs is not itself counter to patients' interests. Even when hospital bills are completely covered by insurance, on a macroeconomic scale, patients still benefit from reducing costs. This is because costs are ultimately passed on to consumers and taxpayers so, eventually, we all pay the bill. However, when a hospital cuts costs, do we, as consumers, share in the savings? Lower costs of care should translate into lower costs to insurers, which should translate into lower premiums or at least avoid premium increases. However, the evidence that this kind of trickle-down economics works in healthcare is lacking. For example, health-care spending in relation to GDP was relatively constant between 2010 and 2019 at 17–18%; however, data from the US Bureau of Labor Statistics indicate that, after adjusting for inflation, insurance premiums increased 45.5% over that same period. Thus, there is little evidence that spending less on care benefits patients, at least those paying for private insurance. Whether we, as a society, will ultimately benefit from lower cost of care or whether benefits will be realized mainly by hospitals is an open question. One thing is for sure, however, any harm resulting from lower cost care will be exclusively borne by patients; therefore, patients should have a say in cost cutting.

What other industry would be allowed to operate this way? Healthcare is a service, yet most other segments of the service industry operate very differently. Healthcare is often compared to the airline industry, particularly when discussing safety, and yes, it's true that air travel is, on average, much safer than going to the hospital. In recent years, many of the industrial engineering practices that make air travel safe have been implemented in hospitals, including checklists and mandatory time-outs for various procedures. Getting the wrong leg amputated should be a "never event," and it's getting there thanks to these kinds of practices. However, no one is holding up the airline industry as an example of great customer service. Indeed, most of us who need to travel regularly consider a great flight as one that arrives on time. Comfort, food, and in-flight entertainment have all sunk so low in the last two decades that we rarely expect to enjoy any of it. However, some of this is a direct result of customer purchasing habits. Basic economy is a "thing" after all because that ninety-dollar flight to Las Vegas for the weekend is appealing to enough people. Or to turn it around, if everyone was willing and able to pay for first class, there wouldn't be an economy section.

Now imagine that the airline industry worked like healthcare. Imagine that we didn't buy airplane tickets directly but instead bought insurance to cover an expected trip from Los Angeles to Sydney. The airlines would then decide what kind of flight experience we were going to have based mainly on their expectations of profit and what kind of competition they were facing. Competition should help keep prices low, but there's a catch: you can only use an airline that your insurance company approves, *and* your insurer has secretly negotiated a price with this carrier and is under no obligation to tell you about it. Of course, your insurance company is also trying to maximize its profits, so you can be pretty confident that you won't be flying first-class. You might anticipate all of this and think you are beating the system by buying an insurance plan that guarantees first class. The trouble is that in this bizarre business arrangement, you won't actually find out what first class means until the flight. You may find out that you'll be sitting on a hard seat and eating off-brand potato chips for your fifteen-hour flight. Finally, you might choose to forget about the insurance altogether. You're not planning any trips to Australia after all. However, if you then find yourself having to make the journey, you will not only be at the mercy of the airlines for the conditions of the flight but also for how much they charge, and you won't actually find out how much until after you take the flight. If this all sounds crazy to you, you may be getting some idea of what it feels like to have a major health crisis and deal with our health-care system.

Various solutions have been proposed, and I'll explore these in more detail in chapter 9, but for now, let's just focus on the alignment. How do we get hospitals to be motivated, monetarily or otherwise, to do things that are in our best interests? In other words, how do we create a system where hospitals' interests are aligned with patients' interests? A good place to start is to ask what patients want.

In 2021, Accenture Health and Life Sciences Experience Survey consulted nearly twelve thousand people in fourteen countries. The survey found that patients aren't satisfied being treated in a one-way, one-size-fits-all transaction. They want care that is tailored to them, and their four most important expectations were emotional support, convenience/accessibility, transparency/data security, and fairness. It's pretty clear that our current system fails miserably on these last two. Our system could not be less fair or less transparent. Data security has also been a problem for almost all major hospital systems. What about convenience and accessibility? Hospitals are motivated to bring about improvements in this category, and the growth of telemedicine and other alternative access models such as urgent care centers and community surgery centers are prime examples. Unfortunately, these models tend to work against the first expectation for more compassionate care and emotional support. Interactions with previously unknown providers in person or by phone or video makes emotional support more challenging to deliver effectively. Moreover, it's unclear how any of these expectations will be met more often under a value-based health-care model. None of these features are likely to significantly impact survival (or, in the parlance of cost-effectiveness, the number of quality-adjusted life years for a patient); hence, these features may not be seen as valuable even though these are clearly features that patients desire.

Importantly, hospitals are not the only part of the US health-care ecosystem that is grossly misaligned with customer values. There are numerous parasites that extract dollars from the system but offer dubious benefits. These "middlemen" buy drugs and supplies from wholesalers and sell them back to hospitals or the public at often significantly inflated prices. One such category is pharmacy benefit managers or PBMs. These are the middlemen in the prescription drug benefits department. Employers directly or through their health insurance company hire a PBM to manage the pharmacy benefits for their employees. PBMs buy drugs wholesale and then charge employers often at exorbitant markup. Because fees, discounts, and rebates affect the prices PBMs pay for drugs, it's usually impossible for employers to know the difference between what they are being charged and what the PBMs actually paid for each drug. Perhaps not too surprisingly, as we saw how private health insurers jumped on Medicare Advantage and turned it into a hugely profitable system (for them), health insurance companies are now getting into bed with PBMs and even own them in some cases. UnitedHealth Group owns a large PBM (Optima X). Cigna owns Express Scripts, and CVS Caremark is owned by Aetna. These three companies control approximately 80% of the US market according to the Health Industries Research Center, which provides market research and analysis in the managed care and pharmaceutical industries. As a result, these large PBMs manage pharmacy benefits for most Americans.

Fortunately, after years of inaction, Congress has finally started to focus on this problem. On May 23, 2023, the House Committee on Oversight and Accountability held a hearing titled "The Role of Pharmacy Benefit Managers in Prescription Drug Markets Part I: Self-Interest or Health Care?" At the hearing, members and witnesses highlighted how PBMs have an oversized role in the pharmaceutical marketplace and push anticompetitive practices that undermine patient health and drive up the cost of prescription drugs. Both Republicans and Democrats stressed that there must be greater transparency in the PBM industry and that Congress must address PBMs' harmful tactics. A press release noted that "the Oversight Committee will continue to examine PBM practices to inform legislative solutions that can greatly benefit patients and reduce drug costs." And there is good reason to believe that costs are significantly inflated by PBMs. According to an analysis reported in the *Journal of the American Medical Association* in 2018, due to PBMs, twelve of the twenty most commonly prescribed drugs involved overpayment rates above 33%. The analysis found that among 9.5 million claims, 2.2 million (23%) involved overpayments. Overcharging on generic drugs was significantly more common than brand-name drugs although overpayments were significantly larger on brand-name drugs ($13.46 on average compared to $7.32). Aggregate overpayments totaled $135 million for 2013 or $10.51 per covered member.

Another example of misaligned middlemen is group purchasing organizations or GPOs. These companies buy supplies from manufacturers and sell to hospitals. GPOs began as a way to bring lower costs to hospitals by bulk purchasing, the same way that PBMs came about. However, like PBMs, GPOs have a grossly misaligned business model. Or rather, over time, many GPOs have manipulated the marketplace to maximize profits and pass the costs to hospitals who directly pass them to patients. A popular method used by GPOs is charging manufactures to place their products in their offerings. A manufacturer who refuses to pay the fees can have a hard time selling to hospitals. Conversely, a manufacturer who pays the fees will need to increase what it charges hospitals to maintain its profit margins. When a hospital claims to pay a grossly inflated price for a minor medical device or supply, it is common to blame the manufacturer. One can easily assume that these companies overcharge hospitals, but it may also be that the source of the inflated prices is the excise tax levied by the GPO.

GPOs may also offer manufacturers another benefit: sole-supplier agreements. For a hefty price, the manufacture can become the sole-supplier of a particular product, effectively creating a micro-monopoly within the GPOs' catalogue. In addition to the obvious implications of price manipulation, these arrangements have another dangerous consequence. A sole-supplier arrangement creates a fragile supply chain. When there is only one supplier for all the syringes a hospital uses, a critical shortage can occur when that supplier's manufacturing plant is compromised. Antitrust lawsuits have begun to emerge over GPOs as just four control most of the market share. According to the US General Accounting Office, the two largest GPOs account for approximately 66% of total GPO purchasing nationwide.

Obviously, healthcare in America has become a tangled web of organizations with misaligned business models, many with dubious ethics. Few Americans have any knowledge of many of these organizations and would be shocked to learn the extent of the profiteering that many engage in. Congress, for its part, is just catching up as well, and that's a particularly stark fact in light of proposed overalls in healthcare. What corruption is waiting around the corner for us as we move into the murkier waters of value-based healthcare? How much confidence can we have that the implications of these new models have been well-thought-out, given the obvious deficiencies in the current system that have been allowed to flourish for decades?

CHAPTER 3

How Did We Get Here?

*All the incentives are toward less medical care, because the
less care they give them, the more money they make.*

—John Ehrlichman, Nixon White House Transcripts, 1971

In the traditional doctor-patient relationship, the doctor is viewed as an advocate for the patient. Indeed, in US society, doctors were once viewed with reverence rivaled only by clergy and, in some cases, beyond clergy. Between 1969 and 1976, the American medical drama television series *Marcus Welby, M. D.* aired on ABC, starring Robert Young as the title character. Welby was a kind, avuncular family practitioner who made house calls and was on a first-name basis with his patients. The series was immensely popular, especially for the first three seasons, and was the first program in ABC's history to become the number one show on television. Members of the American Academy of Family Physicians served as technical advisers and reviewed each script for medical accuracy. As such, the show's popularity may have come from its candid and authentic medical content. However, Welby's character was a large component of the show's appeal. For more than a generation, Welby was a stereotype for an independent-minded physician who stridently put his patients' needs first, often using unorthodox methods. Today, Welby would be seen as overly paternalistic and a bit too cavalier. But at the time, he was seen as rather heroic. One can imagine him fighting hospital protocols designed to save money if they were not in his patients' best interest.

Even today, many physicians see themselves as fighting for patients. Most physicians reject the notion that a patient is a client or customer and with good reason. The obligations physicians have historically accepted by acting as "health-care providers" go well beyond the typical vendor-customer relationship. The Hippocratic Oath compels physicians to "first do no harm," and the implicit extension of this edict is to always act in the patient's (not the doctor's or the hospital's) best interest. Even the interest of society as a whole takes a back seat to the individual patient. This is best illustrated by the use (or overuse) of antibiotics where physicians are reluctant to risk undertreating patients (a threat to the individual) even though overuse of antibiotics results in resistant organisms (a threat to society at large).

Physicians who deal in phony treatments are branded as charlatans and quacks and can face disciplinary action by medical boards or even criminal penalties. It doesn't matter if the therapies are popular among patients who may willingly pay what is charged. There is an expectation that physicians will practice sound medicine and not simply profit from selling their services. An extreme example would be prescribing medications for profit. Physicians lose their licenses to practice and are imprisoned should they be convicted of selling prescriptions. By contrast, in a typical vendor-customer relationship, if the customer is happy, all is well. By year-end 2021, medical boards in twelve states had already taken action against physicians who were spreading false or misleading information about COVID-19. Compare this to the same misinformation being spread by entertainers, politicians, and journalists. Simply put, physicians are held to a much higher standard by the community at large and, indeed, by the law itself.

This is not to say that profiteering in medicine doesn't happen. In fact, a form of it is quite widespread. Some estimates deem as much as 20% of medical spending as unnecessary, whether it's unnecessary testing or even unnecessary procedures. Sometimes the procedure itself is necessary, but the way in which it's performed adds unnecessary costs, such as using imaging to guide a biopsy needle when the target is readily visible to the naked eye or performing a surgery under general anesthesia when a local nerve block would do. Another common "scheme" is to do procedures that should be bundled as staged procedures.

In his book *The Price We Pay: What Broke American Health Care—and How to Fix It*,[1] Marty Makary, MD describes numerous abuses to the system that he and others have identified using data that compares physician practices on a national scale. In some ways, it's reassuring that only a small number of physicians are "outliers" to generally agreed on standards for ethical practice. Given that the system itself often creates huge financial incentives for physicians to

---

[1] Marty Makary, MD, *The Price We Pay: What Broke American Health Care—and How to Fix It* (Bloomsbury Publishing, 2019).

behave in unethical ways, it's reassuring that most do not. However, why do we have a system that permits, never mind encourages, any physicians to behave unethically? Importantly, hospitals often encourage these practices as well because they too may benefit from them.

When each of my parents needed surgery, I knew full well that the surgery would bring in more money to both the hospital and the surgeon than a nonsurgical option. I was quite candid with my family about the inherent conflict of interest, and it factored into my opinions about the best course of action. Ultimately, I advised in favor of surgery in both cases but not before independently investigating nonsurgical options. The reality, though, is that it is relatively easy, especially for me as a physician, to evaluate the surgical and nonsurgical options based on the medical literature and not have to rely exclusively on the information provided by the surgeon.

Even if I were not in medicine, I could reasonably seek out this information though it would be much more difficult. However, I have no idea whether the surgeons or the hospitals used less-expensive or less-effective drugs or devices in the process. I have no idea what, if any, corners they may have cut and whether any of these decisions were in my parents' best interest. Neither I nor my parents would have been consulted about the type of anesthesia, pain medication, and surgical equipment or hardware that was used and whether it was most appropriate. I, like everyone else, trusted in the system to do what was best. But can we really trust a system that has created an incentive to undermine care? Do we really believe that the best therapies will be used when hospitals are given a financial incentive to use less-expensive alternatives even if they are inferior?

Of course, physicians don't share in this conflict of interest… or do they? Throughout this book, I've given examples of how physicians are very much part of the problem, either with our consent, purchased or otherwise, or against our will by way of threat or coercion. If this sounds harsh, consider what it would be like to be a young physician working for a medical center. Your employer wants you to do something that is legal and may not even be wrong, but you are convinced that it's not the best choice for the patient. You know that opposing the will of the hospital is going to work against you, and you also know that you have a couple hundred thousand dollars in student loan debt hanging over you. The pay is good at this hospital, and besides, there is only one health-care system in town. Quitting or having your contract not renewed will mean starting over somewhere else. While this situation isn't that different from many other careers, it highlights the fact that when the hospital employs the physician, it has enormous influence over his or her medical practice so any financial conflict of interest that the hospital has is, by point of fact, shared by its employees.

Not long ago, most physician practices were independent. However, in America, the majority of doctors no longer own their practices. Over the last two decades, hospitals have undergone a steady transformation. Large corporations, often arising from successful hospital systems, have gradually acquired other hospitals, effectively eliminating competition in many markets. When smaller community hospitals are taken over by these corporations, there is a shift in priorities away from what's good for the community toward what's good for those who control the reins of power in the corporation.

A messy complication for large hospital systems was that most physicians didn't actually work for the hospital and, in fact, could admit their patients to any hospital they liked. Hospitals granted "admitting privileges" to doctors typically based only on the physician's credentials and possibly some criminal background checks and malpractice claims information. Hospitals were at the mercy of physicians because they, not the hospitals, controlled the flow of patients and, hence, controlled the most important determinant of hospital revenue. As corporations began to control hospitals, business-savvy leadership recognized the flaws in such a system, at least from the hospital's perspective. An obvious solution was to bring physicians and their patients into the system.

Throughout the 1990s and early 2000s, hospitals aggressively purchased physician practices. Something that is still continuing today. Physicians, for their part, often found an unprecedented windfall in the sale of their practices. There were significant downsides, of course, but for many physicians, the cost was acceptable. For physicians in the latter part of their professional lives, they could effectively retire early and passed the consequences of their transaction to the next generation of physicians. For younger physicians, there were also advantages, such as having a more predictable income and schedule. Corporate control came with benefits that many younger physicians, often struggling with debt, found attractive.

The conflict of interests that became integral to this new arrangement may not have been obvious to physicians at first. However, no physician working for a hospital today is unaware that the system is biased. Well-meaning but unempowered physicians may try to work around the system to get patients what they need while other physicians may actively take part in deceptive practices for a cut of the revenue. It has always been possible for an unscrupulous physician to put their own financial or professional interests ahead of their patients'. What's changed is that it has become very difficult, even for the most conscientious physicians, to consistently put their patients' interest first. Physicians have gradually become complicit in the business of medicine such that they can't break free, and hospitals, intentionally or not, shackle physicians with "golden handcuffs."

Physicians in America earn the highest salaries in the world, yet there are fewer physicians per capita in the US than almost anywhere in the developed world. According to World Bank, there are, on average, 1.8 physicians per thousand people on earth. However, this ratio varies dramatically across countries, from less than 0.1 in many African nations to 8.4 in Cuba. In Europe, Italy has the most doctors, eight for every thousand people, compared to 3.7 in the Netherlands and 3.4 in Ireland. The US only has 2.6. Among high-income countries, only Japan at 2.5 and Canada at 2.4 have fewer doctors per one thousand people. Furthermore, while physicians are increasing sharply in relation to populations in Japan and Canada, they are increasing much more slowly in the US. As such, very soon, if not already, since the World Bank data is running two to three years behind, the US will have the lowest ratio of doctors to population of any high-income country in the world. How do physicians in the US manage? They do so largely because of physician extenders.

In the US, advanced practice nurses and physician assistants provide a lot of the care that only physicians are allowed to deliver in much of the rest of the world. These providers can prescribe medication and perform certain procedures. They function as "extenders" because they are not fully licensed as doctors to practice medicine. Thus, physicians supervise the care they provide, often only loosely, and because they are paid less than half of what physicians are paid, they effectively allow for physicians to earn higher salaries—and, you guessed it, hospitals to pay a bit less in overall clinician salaries. In the US, there are over half a million licensed physician extenders (including nurse practitioners, physician assistants, and nurse anesthetists); therefore, if they were counted as doctors, the ratio of doctors to population in the US would be closer to four per thousand and more on par with the rest of the developed world. Since these physician extenders are often employed by the hospital, they represent another means of control over physician practice. In essence, the hospital holds all the cards. They pay the physician a handsome salary and benefits, and they provide help in the form of physician extenders. In this way, they ensure that physicians will do almost anything they are asked to do.

This is not to say that physicians will violate their professional standards just to appease their employers or even that most employers will ask them to do things that are against the standard of care. Most physicians do hold themselves to a high level of professional accountability, and most hospitals are not so completely focused on dollars that they would force clinicians to do things that are clearly wrong. However, the game is played with significantly more nuance. Most hospital administrators don't see themselves as cheating patients. In fact, most see themselves as champions for quality. Not quality at any cost, though—hospitals strive for "value."

Long before the term *value* became a buzzword for hospitals, there was a significant outcry about the growing cost of US healthcare. Throughout the 1970s, hospital spending grew at a staggering 14% per year, outpacing GDP by 5%. In 1971, the same year Marcus Welby, MD hit the top of Nielson ratings, President Richard Nixon had a meeting with his friend Edgar Kaiser at the White House. During the meeting, Nixon expressed his support for the concept of managed care, which, according to official transcripts, John Ehrlichman, White House counsel and domestic adviser, described as: "All the incentives are toward less medical care, because the less care they give them, the more money they make."[2] Although Kaiser Permanente disputes this description and notes that various briefs were proved to Ehrlichman and the White House that describe it more fairly, the description nonetheless serves to illustrate an essential truth: that managed care was and is about saving money by doing less. So much money, it seems, that some could be siphoned off to incentivize health-care providers while still being advantageous to insurers.

Kaiser Permanente is also an important example, indeed, one of the first and best-known examples of an integrated delivery system (IDS). Kaiser is comprised of three segments: Kaiser Foundation Health Plans, Inc., Kaiser Foundation Hospitals, and the Permanente Medical Groups. The three groups cooperate under mutually exclusive contracts to provide one-stop health-care services.

Although Kaiser is a well-liked system by patients, routinely achieving high patient satisfaction for all three arms of the organiza-

---

2   Richard Nixon, "Transcript of Taped Conversation between President Richard Nixon and John D. Ehrlichman (1971) that led to the HMO act of 1973."

tion, an IDS is fundamentally lacking in the usual checks and balances that we used to associate with healthcare. Specifically, insurance companies serve to check the power of hospitals to set charges; physicians fight insurance companies to provide benefits to their patients; while hospitals check the power of physicians through a variety of methods such as pharmacy and therapeutics committees and physician privileging. While certainly far from perfect, this tradition serves to oppose the concentration of power among any of the three groups. At least, in theory, these checks can serve the interest of patients. Physicians advocate for their patients to receive the best treatments; insurance companies control costs, which, in the aggregate, at least, can hold down premiums; and hospitals can help ensure best practices among its physicians. An IDS subverts these checks and balances, and Kaiser and organizations like it have full control over what drugs they use, what staffing ratios are maintained in the hospital, and what they pay their staff. In turn, patients are at the mercy of the system with just the sort of potential conflicts of interest that we have been discussing in this book, except that it's all one organization.

In German, the word "kaiser" means "king" or "emperor," and just like a benevolent king may rule in the best interest of his people, there is nothing to ensure that he does. Historically, most kings have put their own self-interests ahead of their people. As more IDSs emerge, and there are now many, the potential for profiteering while flying the flag of cost containment is great.

This idea appears central to virtually all innovation in US health economics, creating incentives for providers to do less, meaning they spend less, pocketing the difference. By presetting what payors will pay for a particular treatment, overall costs can be controlled, and setting these payments at a rate that allows hospitals to still spend less ensures that some profit will be made. Ehrlichman's observation from a half-century ago that incentivizing providers to do less would lower costs still motivates thought processes in health economics today. IDSs make such processes more efficient but, at the same time, more susceptible to manipulation. Breaking up IDSs would add a much-needed check on concentrated power. The problem we are now facing, though, is that controlling health-care costs has become the prime directive within government. Safety always increases costs. Airbags add between three thousand dollars and five thousand dollars to the price of a new car. Eventually, our cost-only focus on healthcare will cause enough harm to patient outcomes that our focus will shift. It's unfortunate that there doesn't appear to be an airbag argument for healthcare.

Although the "value-based" health-care delivery model implies that providers, including hospitals and physicians, are paid based on patient health outcomes, implementation of these models focuses mainly on cost. The use of the term "value" in this context is interesting in itself. According to the *Oxford English Dictionary*, "value" is "the regard that something is held to deserve; the importance, worth, or usefulness of something." Most of us would put our health and, indeed, our survival at a pretty high value. We also value comfort and convenience, but are these aspects being included in value-based health-care models? I will discuss this in more detail in chapter 5, but for now, the simple answer is not yet. It remains to be seen just what value (and whose values) are considered. What value really means in the context of healthcare is "economic value"—the amount (of money or goods or services) that is considered to be a fair equivalent for something else. If this definition appears subjective, it most decidedly is. What is the economic value of your health? Of your comfort or convenience? Who's to say?

In the end, value-based models are set to deliver care, which is judged equivalent to care under another model for a lower price. Under such an analysis, if the care is standardized, a lower cost equates to a higher value and a higher cost to a lower value. In other words, something that doesn't change the quality of care is judged to be lower value if costs are higher and higher value if costs are lower. This sounds pretty objective, but evaluating quality of care is often very subjective.

Let's say that you need treatment for a heart condition, and treatment options for this condition include various medications, medical procedures, and even surgery. Let's say that treatment A results in equivalent survival and quality of life compared to treatment B. Are the treatments equivalent? Suppose treatment A results in an 80% patient satisfaction while treatment B only 20%. How do we assign a monetary value to this difference? To make matters worse, our estimates of quality of life and even survival have some uncertainty around them. No two patients are exactly the same, so comparison of survival needs to adjust for variables that affect survival apart from the care itself. Even the best adjustment can only estimate the true effect. So if I tell you that treatment A has a survival rate of 80%, and treatment B is 75%, both after adjusting for patient variability in a sample size of one thousand people, I might conclude that the two treatments are equivalent at least in terms of survival. Therefore, if treatment B was less expensive, even by a small fraction, I would determine it to be of greater value. But is this really true? Later in this book, we'll examine how hospitals, insurers, and government use statistics not just to estimate differences in treatment effects but also to justify business practices.

A rather arbitrary 95% probability is most often used to determine if a difference is "real" or by chance. If we were to determine that there is only a 90% probability that treatment A was superior to treatment B, we would judge that they are not "statistically different." However, if I told you that treatment A has a 90% probability of being even slightly more likely to result in survival, I'm betting you'd be willing to pay something more for it. How much more would likely reflect your financial means but possibly also other variables? For example, if treatment A requires you to be uncomfortable for twice as long as treatment B, you might view a slight difference in survival as less critical.

When my son suffered a broken jaw, he was given two options: Option A was associated with a greater likelihood of success but required that his jaw be wired shut for a few weeks. Option B was slightly more dicey (a small but statistically significant difference in failure rates) but only required that he be on a soft diet. He was offered both options, and because he was nearly an adult, we let him choose. However, if option B were to cost more, and it very well might have, a hospital could decide that it would only offer option A because "results were statistically better." Such a decision would be defensible under a value-based model, but it would not have considered my son's preferences. Since ultimately, I was responsible for the costs in this case through insurance premiums paid over many years, shouldn't I have a say in this? Or be able to give my son a say?

Even if there is no dispute about the relative value of various aspects of care, for example, if a treatment is better in terms of success rates and patient satisfaction, how do we determine its value over another treatment? Over time, medical practice is expected to advance. If something is a little better by all objective measures, when do we decide that it's worth a higher price, and how much higher?

Value-based models currently lack such sophistication and operate best when there is no change in treatment effectiveness. They seem to be predicated on medicine staying stagnant and alternative therapies having no net benefit. In such cases, cost is the only deciding factor. If something is better, there are methods to analyze its relative value, and this can help determine whether the benefits warrant any added expense. We'll tackle the science behind this sort of decision-making in chapter 8, but here I just want to make the point that behind all forms of managed care are explicit assumptions about the relative benefits, or lack thereof, for various treatments. As anyone who has dealt with a medical problem well knows, our opinions as to the value of various benefits (and avoidance of harm) can vary greatly from person to person.

Although earlier forms of prepaid healthcare existed in the US as early as the turn of the twentieth century, the modern health maintenance organization (HMO) didn't emerge on any scale until the 1950s, and even then, they were uncommon and quite small. Prior to Nixon's meeting with Edgar Kaiser, there were only about forty HMOs in existence. However, the Health Maintenance Organization Act of 1973 changed things. This act had three main provisions: (1) Grants and loans were available to start or expand an HMO; (2) Federally certified HMOs were exempt from various state-imposed restrictions; and (3) Employers with twenty-five or more employees were required to offer HMO options. This final provision expired in 1995, but not before it helped establish a foothold for HMOs in the employer-based market.

As prepaid healthcare, the business model of an HMO is to pay for clinical services from providers and hospitals in advance, shifting any economic risk to hospitals and clinics and ensuring a fixed margin for the HMO in exchange for a steady revenue stream for the providers. However, the nature of potential conflicts of interest changes with this arrangement. Because the hospital or clinic is contracted to be paid a fixed sum for a specific number of patients, there's no incentive to provide unnecessary care because revenue is fixed. However, there *is* an incentive to provide less care. Ehrlichman's depiction of incentives being aligned toward less medical care is exactly the point. If one believes that the problem with US healthcare is too much care, then HMOs offer a solution; if we believe that the problem is too little, then it's the exact wrong approach. Of course, the reality is that the problem with US healthcare is both. Neither too much nor too little healthcare is aligned with patients' interests.

If we have a meal at a restaurant and are served dishes that we didn't order but are nevertheless expected to pay for, we're unlikely to be satisfied. Indeed, most of us would be pretty upset. However, if the solution we are offered is to pay a fixed price that we agree on up front but receive less food or lower quality food than we were expecting, we'll likely be no happier. Interestingly, though, if we are paying the bill for a complete stranger and we are offered these two options, more than what was ordered at a higher price or less than what was desired at a lower price, we might find it easier to decide.

In essence, this is the arrangement most of us have with our private or government insurers. To them, a cost savings is a cost savings, at least until we are angry enough to do something.

A final point is that after all of this, it's not even clear that HMOs lower costs compared to traditional insurance. Although out-of-pocket costs are reduced for consumers, controlling for other factors, HMOs may not affect total expenditures and payments by insurers. Some analysts have asserted that HMOs actually increase administrative costs and tend to cherry-pick healthier patients. It may simply be that the profit motive is just a poor fit for medical care. Alternatively, "profit" may not be the best word. "Greed" might be more appropriate.

In his January 2023 editorial in the *Journal of the American Medical Association*, Donald Berwick, MD, a seasoned health-care reformer, writes: "The grip of financial self-interest in US health care is becoming a stranglehold, with dangerous and pervasive consequences."[1] Berwick argues that greed, not fair profit, is at the root of the US health-care crisis. He makes the point that a vicious cycle has evolved in which "unchecked greed concentrates wealth, wealth concentrates political power, and political power blocks constraints on greed." He advocates for health-care professionals to speak out about the harm that excessive private gain and emphasis on profit are doing to patients.

I agree with his concerns, many of which are expressed in this book. However, we also need to acknowledge that we, as health-care professionals, have become complicit in the system of greed and have

---

[1] DM Berwick, "Salve Lucrum: The Existential Threat of Greed in US Health Care," *JAMA*, (January 30, 2023).

accepted a role as hospital fiduciary in direct conflict with our professional role and duty to our patients. As dysfunctional as our government can be, our system of checks and balances was put in place precisely to oppose the concentration of power in one branch. By bringing the three "branches" of healthcare (doctors, hospitals, and insurers) under one administrative unit, we have introduced infinite potential for corruption and removed all reasonable safeguards. Restoring checks and balances to our health-care system is essential to solving the crisis and disrupting the vicious cycle of unchecked greed.

CHAPTER 4

The "Big Lie" in Healthcare

You'll bankrupt the hospital.

—Anonymous

More than one thousand US hospitals closed in the latter half of the 1970s alone, a trend that continued, albeit at a slower rate, throughout the 1980s and into the early 1990s. A report by the Office of Inspector General detailed 440 closures of short-term, acute care hospitals in the decade ending in 1999. While changing demographics from region to region might explain some closures, only seventy-eight new hospitals opened over the same period, so 362 net hospitals were lost over the period. Furthermore, hospitals were also getting smaller. In 1975, there were nearly 1.5 million hospital beds in the US; by 2015, that number had fallen to less than nine hundred thousand.

Prior to the COVID-19 pandemic, the financial health of US hospitals was already in question and the subject of numerous editorials and analyses. One metric is the operating margin; another is cash on hand. The *operating margin* is simply the difference between revenue and expenses expressed as a percentage. So, for example, if a hospital has revenues of one hundred million dollars and expenses of eighty million dollars, the margin is twenty million dollars or 20%. Most hospitals in the US run an operating margin under 2%, and many, particularly rural hospitals, run less than 1%. Even hospitals with a top credit rating (AA+) averaged operating margins of only 4.5% in 2020 according to S&P Global Ratings report. *Cash on hand* is the total liquid assets available to a business, and for hospitals, this is usually expressed as the number of days a hospital could operate without any revenue. For most US hospitals, this number is less than 365 or less than a year of cash on hand. However, both of these indices are potentially misleading. Hospital operations are complex and fluid. What hospitals count as expenses and when they count them can significantly impact the operating margin.

Hospitals buy real estate and capital equipment. They stockpile supplies and pay bonuses to employees. They often engage in activities outside their core operations, such as community surgery centers, urgent care centers, and rehabilitation facilities. Acquiring and running these assets affect their operating costs. In short, there are a number of variables that influence a hospital system operating margin, and many are within its control to manipulate.

In August of 2022, according to public disclosures, Kaiser Permanente reported over $23.47 billion in total operating revenues, representing a small (0.9%) drop from the second quarter of 2021. Total operating expenses were also up slightly (0.2%) to $23.38 billion. The result was an operating income of $89 million (0.4% operating margin) during the second quarter of 2022, down from the prior year's \$349 million (1.5% operating margin). At one level, it may look as though the organization is struggling, but a mere 1% change in expenses, something an organization can almost always achieve, would have created an entirely different narrative.

Similarly, expressing an organization's cash on hand in terms of days can be very disingenuous. If an organization has four hundred million dollars in annual operating expenses and only two hundred million dollars in cash, it could say that it has only 183 days' worth of cash on hand. However, this suggests that if hospital revenues suddenly stopped, the hospital could only survive six months. First of all, cash on hand is only one measure of a hospital's assets, and usually, it's the least robust. Hospitals often have investments, endowments, and real estate assets as well. It's like saying that you're nearly broke because you only have a few hundred in cash and only a few thousand in your checking account while possessing millions in stocks and bonds. Furthermore, in any given year, the hospital can ensure that it only has the cash on hand that it needs and invest the remaining profit in vehicles with higher returns.

But even if we were to look at all the assets a hospital has and express this figure in days, we would still be pretending that a hospital spends just as much when it's empty as when it's full. In fact, if a hospital's revenue were to fall off precipitously, it would be because people stopped coming, and overall operating expenses would decline as well. Sure, some costs are fixed, but most of what a hospital spends money on involves the care of patients, and if there are no patients, costs would be reduced, at least partially. This is precisely what happened during the pandemic. Elective surgery dried up almost overnight. Outpatient services were halted completely and then moved forward at a reduced pace, shifting many services to telemedicine. Hospital administrators panicked, and congress passed a huge relief package to prevent hospitals from going under.

But by the end of the first year of COVID-19, a strange reality became apparent. Many hospitals were showing huge profits even amid the worst of the pandemic. Profit at HCA Healthcare, the country's largest for-profit hospital system, was up considerably, posting a $3.8 billion profit, more than it made in 2019. The company was doing so well that it gave its government relief money back. Tenet Healthcare, another large chain, made almost four hundred million dollars in profit as did several other hospital systems. Interestingly, most kept the government payments, citing future projected losses as the pandemic wore on. However, wealthy hospitals continued to do well. The Mayo Clinic posted $1.2 billion in profits for 2021, a 14% increase from the year before, and its second quarter earnings in 2022 were on track to exceed this for the year. Indeed, elective procedures rebounded sharply in 2021 to 2022 as these cases didn't disappear; they were just delayed.

The situation was quite different for less wealthy hospitals caring for largely uninsured or public insurance patients, so-called safety net hospitals. National Public Radio reported that in October of 2020, the investors' service Moody's warned urban counties that operating a public hospital (most of which are safety net hospitals) during COVID-19 now carried "operational risk." Expenses from personal protection equipment (PPE), staff, and equipment were creating "operating losses," the report said. However, loss projections at large wealthy hospitals, which were shared widely with the media and with hospital workforces, never materialized at many centers.

The pattern isn't new. Since the 1970s, when hospital bankruptcies were getting news coverage coast to coast, hospitals have maintained that they need to continue to cut costs just to stay open. Government agencies and politicians reinforced this idea, citing huge annual increases in health-care spending. But as health-care spending increases leveled off in the 1990s and numbers of hospitals in business stabilized, most hospitals continued to maintain the position that cost containment was a top priority. This is not to say that hospitals were unwilling to spend money. Specialty hospitals, surgical centers, cancer units, and cardiac institutes cropped up all over America, and new ones continue to open today. However, rather than portraying these investments honestly as strategic business decisions to improve profitability, I've heard hospitals argue that even more cost cutting would be necessary in other areas to make these investments and that these investments were required "just so the hospital could survive."

This narrative is the essence of the "*big lie*" in US healthcare; that is hospitals, all hospitals, are "at the brink of insolvency." This is how hospitals can convince their professional workforce that they must hold down costs and endure a variety of austerity measures, the end result of which is that more money is diverted from patient care. If we examine the *big lie* closely, we'll discover that hospital economics is complicated business, and it's no wonder that even healthcare workers have a hard time understanding it. The vast majority of physicians, nurses, and pharmacists working for or with a hospital system have very little direct information on the hospital's finances. They know roughly what the rest of us know when we read the newspapers, and in some cases, this information contradicts what they are being told by the hospital administration.

According to a 2020 report[2], the ratio of health-care CEO pay to average worker pay was 253:1. The top five highest-paid hospital CEOs received salaries between $6.9 and $30.3 million dollars. Furthermore, total compensation, which includes bonuses, is often much higher. According to the same report, the highest-paid health-care executive in 2020 had a salary of $1.6 million, but his earnings were nearly $200 million. Massive executive compensation in health-care, together with high executive-to-worker pay ratios, is exhibit 1 for the *big lie* in healthcare.

The second piece of evidence concerns hospital revenues. According to the US Census Bureau, total revenue for hospitals has been growing sharply for many years. Total revenues for the first quarter of 2005 were $152 billion, increasing to $196 billion by the last quarter of 2009. By the end of 2019, revenues had reached over $300 billion a quarter. Data on health-care spending are less easy to find; therefore, calculating hospital profits can be difficult.

As we've just discussed, we can't rely on measures such as operating margins and cash on hand as these measures are easily manipulated for the hospital's own purposes. If a hospital builds an imaging center, it can call this expenditure an expense in one year and then sell the asset a year later to offset a projected revenue shortfall. Of course, these details will be reported in financial statements; it may still be hard to evaluate the overall financial status of a hospital system without an in-depth analysis. However, by far, the largest costs that hospitals have are for labor. Over the same decade that hospital revenues increased by more than 50%, average physician salaries

---

[2] https://www.beckershospitalreview.com/rankings-and-ratings/the-7-highest-paid-health-system-ceos.html.

increased by only 21%.[3] Now this doesn't necessarily reflect what hospitals paid physicians because 44% of doctors in 2020 were still self-employed, and a decade ago, this figure was 55%. Still, it's one reflection of labor costs.

Another is nursing salaries. Between 2010 and 2018, not quite a decade, median salaries for RNs increased only 11%. If we extrapolate two more years at the same rate of growth, it would still be less than 14%. So if the largest costs that hospitals are wrestling with have increased between 14 and 21% in the same decade that revenues have soared to over 50%, it's reasonable to assume that profits have been increasing, and the *big lie* in healthcare is just that, a *big lie*. However, there is even more evidence that this is exactly the case.

The Federation of State Medical Boards (FSMB) Physician Data Center (PDC) was established in 2004 and regularly receives and analyzes physician licensure data from state medical boards. A snapshot of actively licensed physicians was reported in 2018 and compared to 2010. Over this time frame, there was an increase in licensed physicians of 16% compared to a 6% increase in the US population over the same time frame. However, the age of the US population is increasing, and so is the age of physicians. In 2010, only 25% of physicians were sixty or older. In 2018, that number had increased to 30%. Thus, with an older population requiring more care and an older physician workforce more likely to be working part time, the actual ratio of practicing physicians to patients has likely decreased even while physician numbers have seen some growth.

Another way to look at the problem is to examine national health expenditure (NHE) data. According to an analysis by the

---

[3]   https://money.usnews.com/careers/best-jobs/physician/salary.

Peterson Center on Healthcare, a nonprofit health-care watchdog, hospital spending in the 1970s grew at a staggering 14% per year, outpacing GDP by 5%. This growth eased somewhat in the 1980s but was still nearly 10% per year. However, over the last decade, the annual increase in hospital spending has been under 5%. Thus, even with exorbitant executive salaries, hospital revenues and spending have been closely matched for several years. Importantly, these practices are not restricted to for-profit companies. For example, while Kaiser Foundation Health Plan (KFHP) posted revenues of $58,440,598,902 and expenses of $58,133,304,182 in 2021 (a difference of only 0.53%), they also posted that their top ten salaried executives all made more than two million dollars in compensation (an expense). Interestingly, none of these executives devoted more than twenty-five hours per week, so KFHP paid out more than forty-five million dollars to the top ten earners in its C-suite, and all were essentially working part time! In fact, Kaiser paid forty-five million dollars for 212 hours per week. Assuming a forty-hour workweek, they paid forty-five million dollars for only five and a quarter full-time equivalents or an average of $8.5 million per full-time executive. So, yes, KFHP has a narrow "profit" margin but with top executives all pulling in exorbitant salaries. When excess revenues are distributed to shareholders, we call this a for-profit industry. If the same money is instead distributed to executives, we call this a nonprofit?

Another way to examine hospital finances is to look at hospital systems that are run by publicly traded for-profit companies. Market capitalization, commonly called market cap, is the total market value of a publicly traded company's outstanding shares and is commonly used to measure how much a company is worth. HCA Healthcare (HCA) is the largest health system in the US with over two hundred hospitals. As of May 2023, according to financial disclosures, HCA Healthcare had a market cap of $77.13 billion. This makes HCA Healthcare the fourth most valuable health-care company by market cap in the world and, indeed, among the top two hundred of the world's wealthiest companies of any sort. Furthermore, HCA's market cap has increased steadily over the last decade from a mere twenty-one billion dollars in 2013 to fifty billion dollars in 2019 to more than seventy-seven billion dollars today. Universal Health Services (UHS) is the second largest with 180 hospitals and a more modest market cap of $10.09 billion, nearly double its market cap from a decade ago. Another behemoth is Select Medical (SEM) with 116 hospitals. Its market cap also more than doubled in the last decade from $1.3 billion at the start of 2013 to $3.3 billion at year's end 2022. Thus, according to financial statements, big hospital systems are incredibly profitable and getting more profitable every year.

While siphoning off hospital profits into returns for investors or exorbitant compensation packages for hospital executives instead of improved patient care or lower costs for patients should concern us all, an additional concern is how the *big lie* in healthcare is used to manipulate health-care professionals. Department meetings at hospitals for clinicians used to be about improving care, reducing unsafe conditions, and promoting education. Today, these meetings are often also about furthering the *big lie*. "Hospital revenues are down this quarter, so we need to cut back on the use of the following medications…" "Yes, the operating margins are running well above last year, but we need them even higher so we can obtain a AA+ bond rating or we won't be able to build the new heart institute, and if we can't do that, our competitors will put us out of business." These are not idle conversations. Doctors and nurses on the front lines are fed a steady stream of harrowing accounts of how close the whole system is to collapse. While such tactics are used by many companies to help avert labor disputes, it's only recently become a standard way of operating in US hospitals, and it's not just the employees getting scammed. When the federal government decided to provide preemptive COVID-19 relief to hospitals in 2020, they decided to send out the first forty-six billion dollars in relief money based on how much revenue a hospital had in 2019. What this meant was that the larger the revenue a hospital posted in 2019, the larger its payment was for 2020. But did this make any sense? Large revenues at a hospital might have come from a large elective heart surgery program. Hospitals could simply take the money and shutter the program. There was no requirement that hospitals use the funds on essential services. Meanwhile, poorer hospitals, those less likely to have lucrative cardiac surgery programs or investment portfolios and healthy endowments, received less money because, in fact, they had lower revenues.

It's critical to understand that this is not just about hospitals making excessive profit and paying their leadership excessive compensation. It's also about how this system harms patients. Many books and articles have detailed how predatory hospital billing practices have hurt patients. Just type "predatory hospital billing practices" in your favorite search engine, and you'll be treated to hundreds of hits. Almost everyone in America has or knows someone who has been hit with high medical bills, and many have trouble paying them. The high costs of healthcare, medication, and medical supplies in this country will surprise no one.

However, almost no one talks about the insidious effects of the *big lie* on daily medical practice. In the previous chapter, I outlined various ways hospitals reduce costs by reducing money spent on patients. For some of these, such as cutting staff, the hospital can act unilaterally. But for most, clinicians need to agree. When physicians are led to believe that using a less-expensive therapy, ordering fewer tests, or discharging patients early is vital to the survival of the organization and, by extension, to their own livelihood, they have an enormous conflict of interest. We require physicians to disclose *outside* conflicts of interest when giving presentations to other physicians or publishing in the medical literature. We even have a public reporting database put in place by the Physician Payments Sunshine Act of 2010 so any financial transaction between a pharmaceutical or medical device company and a physician over ten dollars or over one hundred dollars per year in aggregate must be reported. Yet there is no requirement for hospitals to disclose their conflicts of interest when it comes to providing care to patients, nor for physicians to disclose the ways in which their employers require them to practice.

Twenty-three of the nation's largest health-care systems, the majority of which are nonprofit organizations, now have investment arms. These innovation funds or venture capital funds provide financial investment and resources to start-ups in their portfolio. The companies may generate additional revenue for the health system if they are successful. The existence of these funds is additional proof of the excessive profitability of healthcare and yet another potential source of conflicts of interest. Health-care systems are launching ventures in hopes that new technologies will emerge that will generate new revenue streams for their system. But what if that were to happen? What safeguards are in place to ensure that hospitals don't select therapies based on their own intellectual property interests rather than the patients' best interests? Do we really believe that health-care systems should control not only insurance, hospitals, and doctors but now drugs and devices too? Of course, this is entirely consistent with corporate ethos—it's called vertical integration. Some of the same hospital systems that have been created by horizontal integration (business growth by purchasing related businesses, namely, its competitors) are now focused on vertical integration. This is where a business acquires another company to give it greater control over the stages in its supply or distribution chain. Hospitals buying up physician practices could be seen as the first and most disruptive form of vertical integration. Extending this by acquiring imaging centers, laboratories, nursing homes, and rehabilitation centers is the next logical step. No wonder hospital systems have lobbied Congress to roll back restrictions on self-referral (discussed further in chapter 5). It's not to improve value to patients, as is claimed. It's to help them expand and consolidate their business.

It's also important to understand that, increasingly, these are multinational corporations. According to their website, The Mayo Clinic headquartered in Rochester, Minnesota, has offices in fourteen countries, including Canada, India, United Arab Emirates, and multiple South and Central American countries. It also has joint ventures in China and the Middle East. Johns Hopkins has collaborations in more than a dozen countries, mainly in the Middle East but also in China, Japan, and Peru.

One of the first foreign ventures by a US hospital was an organ transplant program in Palermo, Italy, run by a hospital system based in Western Pennsylvania. The venture began in 1997 when Sicily's government and Italian insurers realized it would be cheaper to perform transplant procedures locally than continue to send patients to the US. Since that time, the Palermo facility has performed more than 2,300 transplants. The same health system, one of the most entrepreneurial in the US, also owns hospitals or has had joint ventures in fifteen countries, including Ireland, Italy, China, and even Kazakhstan where they are helping a university develop a medical teaching hospital.

The Cleveland Clinic already has operations in Abu Dhabi and Canada and is now spending nearly one billion dollars to open a hospital across the street from Buckingham Palace Garden. The Mayo Clinic already has a hospital in Central London.

What is the reason for this horizontal integration into international markets? Simple: it's to make more money. Many of the premier health systems in the US have supplemented their revenues for years with wealthy patients coming from abroad. These patients are clearly "out of network" and pay top dollar for services unavailable in their home countries or not available at the same quality. Exact numbers are unavailable, but in some years, the Cleveland Clinic may well have made more money from doing heart surgery on foreign patients than on those from the US.

As early as the 1990s, Pittsburgh was once a prime destination for patients shopping for a liver transplant. The Mayo Clinic offers a suite of "International Patient Services." Their website states: "Every year, patients from more than 150 countries travel to Mayo Clinic for care. International patients receive timely diagnosis and specialty care in a place designed to feel a little more like home." However, nothing feels quite as much as home as home. If you are a Saudi prince, chances are you'd prefer to stay in Riyadh when you need to be hospitalized, and if you do need to travel, wouldn't it be better to travel to, say, Dubai? Indeed, this is exactly what happened. Hospitals offering Western-style healthcare, often with US or European doctors and frequently in cooperation with well-known US entities like Johns Hopkins, began to emerge.

These arrangements are continuing to grow even today. Tawam Hospital and the Johns Hopkins Sidney Kimmel Comprehensive Cancer Center together established a center for specialized medical care and a national referral center for oncology services in the United Arab Emirates. Thus, with greater options for high-priced care closer to home, many US health-care systems started competing with one another right in these markets.

But here, again, the *big lie* in healthcare is alive and well. Writing for Kaiser Health News in 2021, Jordan Rau characterized the situations like this: "Facing the prospect of stagnant or declining revenues at home, about three dozen of America's elite hospitals and health systems are searching with a missionary zeal for patients and insurers able to pay high prices that will preserve their financial successes." I'm not sure where these "prospects of stagnant or declining revenues" are coming from. The data certainly don't support this view. Yet the press seems quite willing to continue spreading the *big lie*. Of course, Kaiser Health News may not be the most unbiased source here, but this story appeared in *The Guardian* and is still available on their website, theguardian.com.[1]

Importantly, as Rau observes, despite their tax designation, nonprofit hospitals in the US are as aggressive as commercial hospitals in seeking to dominate their health-care markets, including internationally, and extract as much money as they can from private insurers. Strangely and in rather stark contradiction to the declining revenue narrative, Rau notes that "some non-profits amass large surpluses most years even as more and more patients are covered by Medicare and Medicaid." He might be on to something.

In over thirty years of practicing medicine, I have found that the vast majority of hospital administrators care about patients and put patients' interests at the top of their priorities. Nurses and doctors work tirelessly for patient safety and to uphold the standard of care. However, our system has been corrupted by corporate interests, and in various ways, it undermines the noble work that these professionals do. Why do we allow such a system to operate unchecked where the only backstop is the consciences of the frontline workers who, increasingly, have their own financial interests intertwined? The *big lie* has served its corporate masters well, and physicians, nurses, politicians, and the press have swallowed it hook, line and sinker.

---

[1] https://www.theguardian.com/us-news/2021/jun/22/us-private-hospitals-europe-cleveland-clinic.

CHAPTER 5

A Closer Look at the Law

That sound you hear is the mingled cheers and exclamations of relief from doctors and other health care professionals across the country as we lift the weight of our punishing bureaucracy from their backs.

—Seema Verma, Centers for Medicare & Medicaid Services, November 2020

As the Trump administration came to a close, CMS (Centers for Medicare & Medicaid Services) announced a historic change in regulations precluding so-called self-referral. The regulations, commonly known as Stark laws, prohibit physicians from referring patients to receive "designated health services" payable by Medicare or Medicaid from entities with which the physician or an immediate family member has a financial relationship. For example, the law prohibits a physician from sending a patient for blood work at a facility that her brother owns or imaging studies in which she has a financial stake. The idea is fairly simple. Much of what a physician orders is at least partially discretionary, and if the physician stands to profit from laboratory or imaging studies or even from a drug that she might prescribe, then it creates a conflict of interest. These restrictions have also been interpreted to limit what facilities a hospital owns. For example, the physicians working for a hospital would not be allowed to discharge patients to a long-term care facility owned by the same hospital. The reason CMS is fighting to roll back these regulations is that they may complicate so-called value-based payment arrangements. Essentially, CMS wants to have an arrangement where an entity is paid to provide care based on outcomes, and it may have trouble implementing such arrangements when multiple entities are involved.

In its November 2020 press release, CMS wrote:

> The old federal regulations that interpret and implement this law were designed for a health care system that reimburses providers on a fee-for-service basis, where the financial incentives are to deliver more services. However, the 21st century American health care system is increasingly moving toward financial arrangements that reward providers who are successful at keeping patients healthy and out of the hospital, where payment is tied to value rather than volume.

Sounds pretty good, doesn't it? As discussed in chapter 2, the business model under which hospitals operate conflicts with patients' interests. These "reforms" to a series of regulations, Stark laws, were designed to eliminate "bureaucratic barriers to value." Proponents argued that with providers taking on the accountability for the total cost of care for their patients, the risks regarding self-referral have changed. The argument is essentially that when a health-care system owns a nursing home and a hospital, transferring a patient from one facility to another is no longer a concern if the organization is paying the bills. In other words, since this arrangement brings in no more revenue, it must be "okay." Indeed, transferring a patient from a hospital to a nursing home could actually be seen as bringing in less revenue, and since costs to a payor (like CMS) would decrease, it could be argued that it brings value to the system. CMS definitely views it this way, stating:

> When we kicked off our Patients Over Paperwork initiative in 2017, we heard repeatedly from front-line providers that our outdated Stark regulations saddled them with costly administrative burden and hindered value-based payment arrangements, said CMS Administrator Seema Verma. That sound you hear is the mingled cheers and exclamations of relief from doctors and other health care professionals across the country as we lift the weight of our punishing bureaucracy from their backs.

The underlying premise of "value-based payment arrangements" is to link payment to patient-centered outcomes. For example, providers can be paid incentives to achieve certain outcomes. This sounds like the answer to the faulty business model discussed in chapter 2.

If a hospital can make more money by achieving outcomes that patients desire, everyone should win. However, what's missing from this description is that value-based care models that have been put forth are motivated first and foremost by saving money. This is why CMS was so exuberant about announcing changes, which, in their words, were aimed at "reducing administrative burdens that drive up costs by taking money previously spent on administrative compliance and redirecting it to patient care." Of course, is it really safe to assume that the same hospital administrators who have been enriching themselves for the last two decades would naturally plough savings from "reduced administrative compliance" into patient care? The smart money would be on "no." To make matters worse, value-based plans have, so far, been entirely unsophisticated. Their most common structure is to provide a lump sum payment for each person covered under the plan and have the provider assume the risk should the patient require more care but profit from the leftover dollars if the patient stays healthy.

The idea is to align the incentives. Patients presumably wish to stay healthy, and if health-care providers can earn a profit on keeping them healthy, everyone wins. However, this model, as anyone who knows anything about medicine or human behavior in general can plainly see, is unquestionably flawed. To call it oversimplistic would be generous.

First of all, the inherent assumption that staying healthy always leads to cost savings, particularly in the short-term, is simply absurd. Sure, there are excellent examples where this is true. If you are a type 1 diabetic, taking your insulin and maintaining an appropriate diet will almost certainly reduce the need for expensive hospital care for life-threatening complications, and it will not take long to see the effect. However, if you are a relatively young type 2 diabetic, complications from your disease may take decades to manifest, and if you are unable to control blood sugars with diet alone, you will require medication. Is it really likely that a provider will be willing to pay up-front costs for the most effective medication now to benefit financially ten or twenty years into the future? Furthermore, new medications might not even be more effective but instead be more desirable because they are easier to take or cause fewer side effects. Will providers consider these benefits when determining what treatments they will make available?

Sure, a value-based payment arrangement for type 2 diabetes could involve maintaining acceptable control of the disease. Providers could be paid, for example, based on keeping patient's hemoglobin A1C, a blood test used to monitor control of diabetes, below a given level known to reduce risks of long-term complications. This would ensure that payments are aligned with patient interests, right? Unfortunately, if the history of the health-care industry is any indication, it may not.

Maintaining hemoglobin A1C is also a function of body mass index (BMI). It would be relatively easy for a system to deny patients with high BMI into this particular value-based payment arrangement. This practice of "cherry-picking" better-paying cases is very common in healthcare and certainly in the playbook used by hospital systems. But it doesn't stop here.

Health systems are investing heavily in artificial intelligence. Some of this investment is designed to improve care by detecting disease earlier or identifying patients likely to respond better to certain therapies. Identifying high-risk patients is a pillar of precision medicine. However, there is no reason that artificial intelligence cannot also be used to identify low-risk patients to place in a value-based payment arrangement. Worse still, when a group of patients is identified who will maintain an acceptable hemoglobin A1C, greater "value" can be achieved by placing them on the least expensive medicine to achieve these goals, even if that means some patients will actually have worse levels or have undesirable side effects.

In the outpatient setting, patients will be told that their value-based care model doesn't cover the more expensive drug. In the hospital, patients will likely not be told anything at all. Hospitals have been playing these kinds of games with our current system. Is there any reason to expect that a corporate health-care leadership will not do the same thing with value-based care models?

Furthermore, if the whole idea behind value-based models is to reduce overall costs, is it really "value-based" at all? And why is it necessary to make sweeping changes in laws that prohibit self-referral to achieve this?

CMS seems to be arguing that Stark laws were put in place to protect the government from being overcharged, and now that government is switching to another means of cost control, value-based payment arrangements, it no longer needs this protection. But were Stark laws really designed to protect the treasury?

The history behind the collection of regulations that are commonly referred to as Stark laws began in 1989 as the Ethics in Patient Referrals bill. The legislation was introduced because of concerns over conflict of interest when physicians refer patients to laboratories that they have a financial stake in. The concern appears to have been well-founded.

A report by the Office of Inspector General concluded that when physicians owned a stake in a clinical laboratory, there was overutilization. In other words, these physicians tended to order more tests. Subsequent studies found similar patterns when physicians owned facilities that performed physical therapy and diagnostic imaging. A 1991 study found that gross and net revenues were 30–40% higher in physician-owned facilities. So, yes, Stark regulations do seem to have been largely motivated by fiscal concerns, but do these really end under a value-based model?

Consider a hypothetical physician-owned imaging center that does mammograms. The management has been considering upgrading its equipment to the latest technology, which we will say is 20% more accurate in detecting breast tumors. If the management knows that reimbursement for the imaging will not increase if they make the investment, the business case under a value-based payment arrangement hinges on whether 20% increased accuracy will influence the value-based outcome and whether it's sufficient to recoup the costs. However, if the management knows that its physician owners will continue to refer patients to the facility either way, the case to upgrade, to add value for their patients, may be less compelling. This would seem like precisely the conflict of interest the Ethics in Patient Referrals bill was intended to address.

There can be no doubt that achieving value for patients is a laudable and important goal. Value-based payment arrangements are being developed to achieve this goal and are intended to address the gross misalignment that has existed in a traditional fee-for-service arrangement. Health-care policymakers are not wrong in their assessment of the problem with our existing system. Regrettably, in medicine, we are familiar with some treatments causing more harm than good. Great care will be necessary in the design and implementation of these models. Otherwise, the cure may be worse than the disease.

Other laws have been enacted in recent years to deal with physician financial conflicts of interest. The Physician Payments Sunshine Act of 2010 was intended to increase transparency of financial relationships between health-care providers and pharmaceutical manufacturers. The legislation requires manufacturers of drugs and medical devices to collect and track all financial relationships with physicians and teaching hospitals and to report these data to CMS. The stated goals of the law are to increase the transparency of financial relationships between health-care providers and pharmaceutical manufacturers and to uncover potential conflicts of interest. The details of the Sunshine Act provisions are incredibly strict. Any financial transaction over ten dollars or over one hundred dollars per year in aggregate must be reported. One observer quipped that a drug company representative could still buy a doctor a cup of coffee, but if he included a biscotti, it would be reportable. While most would agree that there is a public interest in transparency when it comes to physician financial relationships with industry, it seems rather incoherent to track transfers of value as little as ten dollars in a public database while, at the same time, eliminating Stark regulations that could amount to unregulated and undisclosed conflicts involving millions of dollars.

One of the additional consequences of the Physician Payments Sunshine Act of 2010 is that it serves to further a long-held belief among doctors that pharmaceutical companies are inherently evil.

While scandals like those involving opioids are certainly evidence that this impression is true, most pharmaceutical companies do not engage in what amounts to bribes to physicians to sell their products. Still, it's fair to say that a real potential for conflict of interest exists. Importantly, though, doctors are also conditioned to believe that the hospital administration is looking out for them and, in some general way, shares their values to provide the best care to patients. At the very least, most doctors don't expect that their hospital is intentionally shortchanging their patients on healthcare. But as we've seen, that's often exactly what they are doing, and lately, they seem to be getting help from the government as well.

While laws aimed at curbing corrupt business practices in medicine are certainly needed, legislating good medicine is another matter entirely. Indeed, legislators are terrible doctors, even (and maybe especially) the ones who actually are physicians. But even if the legislature was full of eminent medical authorities, the law is a slow, rigid, and grossly impractical way to improve medical practice. Furthermore, as we saw during the COVID-19 pandemic, political interests also drive many efforts as opposed to a genuine desire to foster public health.

For example, when the Tennessee Board of Medical Examiners began to receive complaints that some doctors were relaying fantastical, unsupported claims about the vaccines, including that they magnetize the body, cause infertility, and inject microchips under the skin so the government can track patients' movements, they issued a warning to doctors in the state, advising them that spreading misinformation about COVID-19 vaccines could land them in big trouble with the board, including the possible revocation of their medical licenses. However, the chair of the Tennessee House Government Operations Committee, Republican State Representative John Ragan, determined that the board had overstepped its bounds. Ragan ordered the board to remove the warning from its website and threatened to terminate the board. At the same time, another Tennessee legislator, Republican State Representative Chris Todd, introduced a bill called Tennessee COVID-19 Treatment Freedom Act that would have prevented the board from disciplining any doctor for administering any treatment for COVID-19, even if it "is not recommended or regulated by the department of health, the board, or the federal food and drug administration."

Other states have considered similar legislation. Legislators in half the states have introduced bills that would prevent medical licensing bodies from punishing medical providers who promote COVID-19 misinformation or unproven treatments, according to the Federation of State Medical Boards. So far, only North Dakota has approved legislation—its law protects providers who prescribe or dispense ivermectin—but bills are still alive in many states.

Meanwhile, in California, Democratic Governor Gavin Newsom signed into law AB 2098, a measure that would make it illegal to spread misinformation about COVID-19, defined as "false information that is contradicted by contemporary scientific consensus contrary to the standard of care." However, soon after the law was passed, it was blocked by a federal judge, stating that the measure was too vague for doctors to know what kind of statements might put them at risk of being penalized. "COVID-19 is a quickly evolving area of science that in many aspects eludes consensus," he wrote. Indeed, the American Civil Liberties Union filed briefs supporting plaintiffs in two lawsuits, saying that while the state did have the power to punish doctors for spreading harmful false information, AB 2098 was a blunt instrument that went too far.

Legislators who are pushing to protect doctors from disciplinary action over misinformation say medical boards are interfering in the relationship between patients and their doctors. They say providers should be free to make their own judgments about medical practice. Apparently, though, this only applies to information about vaccines and discredited COVID-19 therapies. Long before COVID-19, politicians at the state and federal levels have sought to meddle in the doctor-patient relationship. In 2011, Florida passed a law restricting physician conversations with patients about guns, a measure described as a physician "gag law" by the *AMA Journal of Ethics*. In various bills at state and federal levels, physician conversations with patients about firearms, abortions, and fracking were subject to restrictions. A similar legislative battle is being waged over gender-affirming treatments, which several states are seeking to prohibit or restrict.

Even when legislation is not politically motivated, it can be deeply problematic. In 2013, New York state imposed Rory's Regulations, named after a twelve-year-old boy who died of sepsis, a severe form of systemic inflammation caused by infection, in a New York hospital. The law is a directive to doctors and hospitals on how to treat sepsis. The key components are rapid diagnosis, prompt use of antibiotics, and aggressive use of fluids.

While a study conducted by Jeremy Khan M.D. at the University of Pittsburgh and published in the *Journal of the American Medical Association* found that the regulations did reduce sepsis mortality in the state, there is still controversy. First, rapid diagnosis almost certainly misdiagnoses some patients. Sepsis rates have been increasing around the world, and mortality from sepsis has been decreasing, but any effort to improve recognition of a disease or condition increases the less severe cases, cases that might have easily been missed. Sure, the law was motivated by the tragic case of Rory Staunton whose diagnosis was initially missed, but the regulations resulted in the identification of many more cases that never would have been identified at all because they were mild and self-limited. Simply counting more of the less severe cases in the denominator will appear to have reduced the mortality rates even if the numerator is unchanged.

Second, while antibiotics sound like appropriate therapy and, indeed, for sepsis, they are, giving more unnecessary antibiotics because of overdiagnosing sepsis will increase the risk of antibiotic resistance, which impacts the population at large. However, the biggest controversy concerns the use of fixed, high volume of fluids, thirty milliliters per kilogram of body weight to be exact.

When the New York law was passed, medical science had a skeptical but somewhat positive view on this volume of fluids based on relatively weak evidence. However, since the law passed, multiple studies, including some of my own research, have questioned the value of this kind of fluid therapy, and some studies have actually shown harm. Thus, it's possible that while some components of the regulations might be beneficial, others may be doing harm. Citing this evidence, the Surviving Sepsis Campaign, a multimedical society-led program to develop and continually update guidelines for sepsis care, downgraded the recommendation for this volume of fluid to a weak "suggestion" in 2021. However, once laws are written, they need to be repealed. There is no mechanism to update the law as medical science evolves. Simply put, legislation will eventually require bad medicine, and even if subsequently repealed, there will be a period of time where the mandate for bad medicine is still in place despite medical science knowing better.

Meanwhile, where regulation is urgently needed, it's absent or being rolled back. Hospitals are not required to disclose their conflicts of interest, their billing practices, or even their rates to patients. Doctors who work at these institutions who are saddled with employer-based conflicts of interest are not required to inform patients, even when outside interests are disclosed down to the ten-dollar level. Programs like Medicare Advantage are enriching insurance companies at great public expense and also take advantage of patients.

There is, of course, another body of law that should be considered in the context of modern US healthcare—antitrust. In various markets, large and small, monopolies exist in healthcare. In small communities, there may only be one hospital available for miles. This problem is not new and can be difficult to address. Creating competition in small markets may not be possible without external manipulation. Traditionally, the idea of a small nonprofit hospital was that it served the community and often was established by donations from the community it was established to serve.

In theory, such a hospital would not require competition to ensure that consumers received maximum value because the mandate of the hospital would be to deliver value, not to make a profit. A board of trustees or similar body would be responsible to represent the interest of the community and oversee hospital management. However, several problems have arisen as the landscape of healthcare in the US has changed. First, many small hospitals in small communities closed in the 1970s, 1980s, and 1990s, forcing patients to use hospitals in other communities and disrupting the relationship between the hospital and the community. A hospital that expanded to serve surrounding communities may not have changed its oversight board to represent those communities, and the mission of the hospital may have become out of step with many of its patients.

A more serious threat is created when a hospital is purchased by another entity. In the extreme case, a small nonprofit is bought out by a large for-profit chain. The new management inherits the *de facto* monopoly but not the public oversight. Often, when this happens, there is a requirement to preserve the public interest in various ways (e.g., proportion of charity care). However, the lack of transparency in healthcare in the US makes monitoring compliance with such mandates difficult. As discussed in chapter 4, the *big lie* in healthcare has created a massive shell game where hospitals can hide revenue and inflate expenses in ways that can obscure their capacity to work toward the public interest.

For example, if a hospital can show a 1% operating margin, might they argue that 1% is as much as they can spend on charity care? Hospitals may also strain credulity when they offer "payment plans" for people who cannot pay and refer to this as charity. If hospitals inflate costs so they exceed insurance and then offer a payment plans so patients can pay the inflated bills over time, that's hardly charity.

Health-care monopolies are not unique to small markets. Hospital systems composed of many hospitals, often in a single region, may capture sufficient market share in a region to be viewed as a monopoly. Importantly, the US Federal Trade Commission (FTC) has been slow in regulating hospital mergers, perhaps because interstate commerce may not be involved. Furthermore, many states have issued Certificates of Public Advantage (COPAs) to hospitals attempting to replace marketplace competition among hospitals with state oversight. Hospitals and some state legislators claim that COPAs help lower costs and improve population health. However, a body of evidence indicates otherwise.

In a press release issued August 15, 2022, the FTC noted research showing that COPAs are often detrimental for patient costs, patient care, and health-care worker wages. "Despite hospital claims that COPAs will result in lower costs and improved population health outcomes, we are not aware of any proven benefits of COPAs," said FTC Director of Policy Planning Elizabeth Wilkins. "We urge state lawmakers to consult local health insurers, employers, and workers regarding the potential impact of COPA legislation."

There is emerging evidence that the FTC is taking a much more aggressive position on hospital mergers and acquisitions under the Biden administration. Biden's executive order on "promoting competition in the American economy"[1] calls on government agencies including the FTC to promote market competition in various industries including healthcare. The president said that hospital mergers and acquisitions had left the ten largest health-care systems in control of a quarter of the market and led to the closure of hospitals in rural and other underserved areas. In response to this order, the FTC

---

[1] https://www.whitehouse.gov/briefing-room/presidential-actions/2021/07/09/executive-order-on-promoting-competition-in-the-american-economy/.

has already blocked some hospital mergers and is considering moves against several other consolidation attempts.

The emergence of integrated delivery systems (IDS) such as Kaiser Permanente and now many others have the potential to manipulate the market in several ways. As discussed in chapter 3, an IDS has the potential to subvert the normal checks and balances that traditionally exist between a hospital, physicians, and an insurer. These organizations have full control over what drugs they use, what staffing ratios are maintained in the hospital, and what they pay their staff. They may create a monopsony. Whereas a monopoly exists when there is only one seller of a given product, a monopsony is where there is only one buyer.

In antitrust, the term is most often used in reference to labor. If there is only one business hiring in a society, then they can manipulate the labor market to affect wages and working conditions. In the context of a hospital system, if every hospital in the region is controlled by a single entity, physicians may feel even more constrained to exercise their professional judgment if it's against the interest of the hospital. Similarly, a hospital might choose to reduce staffing to a level that nurses would quit in a competitive environment but tolerate under a monopsony.

What is clear from recent developments in the US health-care sector is that enforcement of existing laws and perhaps new regulation is urgently needed. Legislatures at the state and federal levels have largely failed to protect health-care consumers. And if recent trends are any indication, it's only going to get worse.

CHAPTER 6

Doctors: Winners or Losers?

*The devil doesn't come dressed in a red cape and pointy
horns. He comes as everything you've ever wished for.*

—Tucker Max

*You load sixteen tons, what do you get?
Another day older and deeper in debt.
Saint Peter, don't you call me, 'cause I can't go.
I owe my soul to the company store.*

—Merle Travis, "16 Tons," Warner Chappell Music, Inc.

The term "physician burnout" was virtually unknown in the US prior to the twenty-first century. This is not to say that burnout didn't occur, but it was not a phenomenon that generated much attention.

In the year 1983, there was only one paper published in the entire medical literature on the topic, and there were never more than fifteen published in any given year until 1991. Even then, publications per year remained in double digits until 2009, a year when there were 118. By comparison, babesiosis, a very rare tick-borne disease had 147 publications in 2009; bubonic plague had 289. Thus, to say that physician burnout, as a topic of scientific study, was a very small niche is probably an overstatement. It follows that there would have been no funding for such research in the late twentieth century and, therefore, no one writing grants to study the problem. The year 2019, the year before COVID-19, changed the landscape of healthcare around the world; there were 781 publications. In 2021, there were 929.

Another term that was unknown just a decade ago is "physician well-being." Today, physician wellness is practically an industry of its own. If you type "physician wellness programs" into your favorite Internet search engine, you will be treated to dozens, if not hundreds, of hits.

In September of 2022, the House Committee on Ways and Means advanced bipartisan legislation authored by four US representatives, three of them also physicians, that would expand access to mental health programs for physicians. The Physician Wellness Program Act (H. R. 8890) would remove barriers that often "prevent physicians from accessing wellness programs." This massive increase in publicity should not be taken as evidence that funding has increased to study the problem, however.

As of 2023, there is no federal funding or support for vital research in clinician well-being. One of the six core recommendations in the 2022 National Academy of Medicine consensus report was for the US to allocate dedicated research funding to advance clinician well-being. The report specifically called on Congress to allocate funding to various federal agencies including the National Institutes of Health and the Department of Veterans Affairs to support this research.

Although research is still lagging, by all accounts, physician well-being is on the decline. Experts studying the problem, presumably in their spare time, point to regulatory requirements, administrative burden, and the clinical practice environment along with many other factors. The COVID-19 pandemic exacerbated the problem in multiple ways. Clinicians in general, not just physicians, experienced hospital mortality and patient suspicion at levels unprecedented in more than a generation. These stresses contributed to staff turnover, which led to major short staffing only exacerbating the problem further. Recent data suggest that nearly one-third of health-care workers experience moderate to severe levels of depression and anxiety and that four times as many have reported severe mental health challenges compared with before the pandemic.[2] Importantly, there is a growing body of evidence that links clinician well-being to patient safety and quality outcomes. Thus, addressing the problem is not just in the interest of physicians but also patients.

Ironically, programs designed to improve the quality and safety of healthcare may actually contribute to poor well-being by overburdening clinicians with additional workload, thus further jeopardizing delivery of high-quality care. A knee-jerk reaction in many industries is to address safety and quality with additional worker training and product surveillance. In healthcare, physicians as workers are sub-

---

[2] J. Gilleen et al., "Impact of the COVID-19 Pandemic on the Mental Health and Well-Being of UK Healthcare Workers," *BJPsych Open* 7, no. 3 (2021): 88. https://doi.org/10.1192/bjo.2021.42.

jected to mandatory in-person or online training exercises (many of which are time-consuming and ineffective) and, at the same time, are required to contribute to "product surveillance" by filling out forms and online instruments to monitor care or, in the extreme, mandate certain practices. Physicians, who are all licensed by the states, have the ability to override such mandates for individual clinical exceptions, but most systems make this option so onerous that doing the right thing for a patient can feel quite hard. Mandatory physician training is almost always an unfunded mandate as well, so clinicians are expected to comply with these requirements on their off-duty hours and for no added compensation.

Physician burnout may also increase the likelihood that a physician will succumb to the temptation to cut corners. A hallmark of burnout is depersonalization, consisting of cynical and negativistic behavior. A burned-out clinician may experience less empathy for his or her patients or simply lack the energy to question superiors about specific care plans. Many aspects of medicine have no clear best answers. Should a physician practicing in a hospital order a test or change a medication? We don't want or expect a finical incentive to be a factor in this decision. We don't want our physicians to put their own self-interests into the equation. Neither do we want the physician to feel apathy and simply do whatever is easiest. We want, in all cases, our physicians to be motivated by doing what is in the best interest of the patients. This not only requires knowledge and clinical judgment but also requires a level of compassion for the individuals and altruism for society as a whole, and these elements may be diminished by burnout. Importantly and perhaps counterintuitively, burnout is not a direct function of workload, nor is it remedied by increased pay.

One other term that has started to appear in articles examining the root causes for the decline in physician well-being is "moral injury." Moral injury refers to social, psychological, and spiritual harm that arises from a betrayal of one's core values, such as justice, fairness, and loyalty. The term has most extensively been used in the context of the actions of soldiers during war but has recently begun to be applied to health-care workers. Harming others, whether in military or civilian life; failing to protect others, through error or inaction; and failure to be protected by leaders, especially in combat—can all wound a person's conscience, leading to lasting anger, guilt, and shame, and can fundamentally alter one's worldview and impair the ability to trust others. In essence, a person who grossly violates what they believe is right may experience persistent self-criticism—feeling unworthy, unforgivable, or permanently damaged. Reflecting on the perceived transgression can fill a person with sorrow and bitterness. More simply, anyone forced to make intense ethical choices risks moral injury.

Moral injury has been identified as a significant contributor to physician stress and burnout. An important consideration is that the violation of a physician's core beliefs doesn't need to be extreme to be impactful. When a patient dies or has another significant adverse outcome, a physician may internalize the outcome as a personal failing. If the physician perceives that the failure was due to lack of knowledge or technical ability, she may seek additional training. If, however, the outcome is believed to have resulted from a failure to provide the best care because the physician is trying to control costs for the system, she may sustain moral injury. In particular, moral injury is more likely when the physician is part of the decision-making. When physicians assume the role of hospital fiduciaries, they risk regretting decisions made for cost over potential benefit. Importantly, there does not even have to be an adverse outcome for physicians to feel that they have compromised their values by going along with cost-containment efforts that put hospital finances and, by extension, their own finances above patient concerns. The cumulative effects of moral injury over time can be devastating to a physician's psyche.

Interestingly, moral injury is rarely addressed in physical wellness programs, and there is a perverse logic to its absence. A large proportion of wellness initiatives are created by or for hospitals, and hospitals are often the source of moral injury for physicians. Thus, the design of a hospital-based physician wellness program may, intentionally or not, fail to mention a major source of the decline in physician well-being.

These high-profile challenges to physician well-being in the US have begun to reverse a century-long trend in physician immigration. According to statistics from the American Association of Medical Colleges, roughly a third of physicians practicing in the US graduated from a medical school outside the US. While some of these physicians may be US born with no intention of ever practicing outside the US, most came to the US to practice medicine. One reason is better pay.

In the US, physicians earn more than anywhere else in the world. Historically, this has led to a brain drain of many of the best and brightest physicians from other countries coming to the US to practice even though these physicians often must repeat years of training to do so.

According to Great Z's anesthesiology blog,[3] in 2020, American primary care doctors made about the same as their German counterparts: $242,000 versus $200,000. But that was still twice as much as primary care doctors made in the UK ($122,000). Furthermore, specialists in the US make roughly 50% more than their primary care counterparts while German specialists actually earn slightly less than German primary care doctors. In the UK, specialists earn $155,000 or only about 25% more than primary care doctors. American doctors make the most money, so as expected, their net worth is far higher. Average net worth of US doctors is $1,742,000 compared to $657,000 in the UK and only $441,000 in Germany.

Importantly, however, average net worth of physicians is misleading when you consider that most physicians begin their careers in debt, and it's only getting worse, such that physicians graduating today will be, on average, in much greater debt than just a decade ago. Unlike in most countries, US doctors carry a huge amount of student loan debt when they graduate from medical school. This expense is carried through the three to seven years of residency and fellowship when there is not enough income to pay back the loans. Indeed, until about twenty years ago, pay to resident doctors was so paltry that many incurred more debt over those years. My salary as a resident in 1988 was just over eighteen thousand dollars a year. By comparison, doctors in many other countries usually train for free or with just nominal fees. Medical malpractice is often either nonex-

---

[3]   https://www.medscape.com/slideshow/2021-international-compensation-report-6014239?src=#1.

istent or a greatly reduced threat outside the US whereas American doctors often face high malpractice insurance expenses.

As a result of these economics, young physicians are usually not in a position to go into private practice on their own and often regard the security of hospital-owned practices quite favorably. A guaranteed salary, benefits, malpractice coverage, vacation, and medical education leave are rather attractive when you are swimming in student loan debt. Commonly, hospitals even offer signing bonuses. By contrast, starting a private practice or even joining an established one means risk. Unfortunately, the "golden handcuffs" of corporate practice come with many unseen and unspoken costs. No one ever asks physicians about their tolerance for moral injury. Indeed, having trained within a hospital system, many physicians probably don't even recognize all the employer-based conflicts of interest. Transitioning from working for a hospital as a resident to working as a fully licensed physician for another or even the same hospital may not seem that significant, having never experienced anything else. In many important ways, training doctors within a hospital system habituates them to accept employer-based conflicts of interest as a fact of life. Soon, in America, we won't have any physicians left who know the difference.

One might then ask a critical question: Are US physicians better off with higher salaries and more debt starting out but greater net worth later on? Does corporate practice with its guarantees offset the reduction in autonomy available in private practice? And do US physicians lament the fact that they are serving the hospital first and their patients second (and are they even aware of this)? One measure could be physician satisfaction.

Even before the COVID-19 pandemic, physician satisfaction in the US has been at an all-time low. In 2016, Medscape, a web resource for physicians, reported results from a survey of more than fourteen thousand US doctors practicing in thirty different specialties about how their work affected the rest of their lives. The results indicated that fewer than half of US physicians were happy at work, and in some fourteen specialties, including cardiology and nephrology, fewer than one-third reported being happy. Happiness was greatest but still less than 50%, for dermatologists and ophthalmologists, two specialties known for better lifestyles than most other physicians. Physician suicide rates are higher than at any time on record, and physicians are leaving the workforce or cutting back in much greater numbers. A 2018 survey found that 54% of physicians were considering retiring in the next five years, including 30% of those under fifty years of age! Sadly, these trends have greatly intensified during the pandemic. A 2021 survey conducted by Physicians Foundation found that 60% of physicians reported being burned out, up from the already extreme rates of 40% in 2018. Worse still, an InCrowd report from Apollo Intelligence found that American physicians experienced more burnout and work-related stress in 2022 than in 2021. According to a press release from InCrowd, there was also a 10% increase in the number of surveyed physicians who considered leaving their profession.

In a 2021 op-ed, Lorna Collier listed seven reasons why physicians are leaving medicine. In addition to burnout, she identified increasing verbal abuse by patients, high debt, insufficient income to pay it, long hours, lack of family time, dealing with hospital bureaucracy and electronic medical records, and reduced autonomy. The connection between these factors and the industrialization of medicine may not be obvious. However, every one of them is a symptom of the disease that has infected American medicine.

Burnout is a function of many factors that I have already discussed, but the constant moral injury that comes from being in the middle of an employer-based conflict of interest is, for most physicians, a significant factor. Verbal abuse by patients is also a symptom as patients increasingly experience frustration over understaffed and under-resourced hospitals. Resident physicians actually work fewer hours now than they did a generation ago thanks to laws passed to reduce the inhumane work hours and the resultant errors in practice that resulted from sleep-deprived doctors. However, if you are also dealing with moral injury and angry patients, the long hours seem far more unbearable. The increase in hospital bureaucracy over the last two decades has been staggering, and at least, some of it is in the service of reducing hospital costs by controlling physician prescribing. The electronic medical record is first and foremost a billing device that is used by hospitals to maximize their reimbursement. Progress notes that we once used to document patient progress and communicate between physicians are now almost exclusively to support billing. And finally, after moral injury, reduced autonomy is perhaps the greatest casualty of the system as it is today. High debt and insufficient income are not related to hospitals *per se,* but medical schools are usually part of health-care systems. Professors at medical schools usually practice medicine in the hospital affiliated with the school. Their compensation is often partly and, in some cases, largely from the medical school, and their clinical work is, in some cases, all but donated to the hospital. If hospitals were less concerned about paying exorbitant salaries to their executives, they could pay academic physicians and perhaps encourage a reduction in the tuition, now more than two hundred thousand dollars. Such a move might help address this last factor, leading to record low physician satisfaction.

Comparing physician satisfaction across countries can be difficult. Satisfaction is tied up in expectations, which vary greatly across countries or even within countries by region, by urban versus rural settings, etc. However, an online survey conducted by Statistica found that US primary care physicians were at the bottom of the eleven countries sampled (Switzerland and Australia were at the top) in terms of physician satisfaction.[1]

In my interviews with physicians working outside the US, further detailed in the next chapter, I found that physician satisfaction is decreasing globally. Reflecting the survey data that I've just presented, most physicians agreed that satisfaction was at an all-time low; and for most countries, the problems began before the pandemic and have now only been further intensified. I could find no physicians anywhere in the world willing to tell me that things are better now than ten years ago. While nostalgia often clouds our perception of how things were in the past, most of us have a pretty good sense of what direction things are going in even if the magnitude is uncertain.

Of the doctors I spoke to in thirteen countries, only those from Thailand indicated similar satisfaction today compared to ten years ago. The exception to this general rule was the VA system here in the US where I found doctors who believed satisfaction was actually higher now compared to ten years ago. This appears to be related to

---

[1]   https://www.statista.com/statistics/1097249/proportion-primary-physicians-satisfied-with-practicing-medicine-select-countries-worldwide/.

a variety of high-profile complaints and criticisms of the VA system a decade ago, and VA doctors now feel that conditions for patients are now dramatically improved. This has greatly increased their sense of satisfaction. Interestingly, whereas doctors in the US, including at the VA, all told me that COVID-19 had a very negative effect on physician satisfaction, this was not true for many other countries.

For example, doctors in Belgium, Brazil, and Thailand all indicated that physician satisfaction was not significantly impacted by the pandemic. Doctors in Spain actually felt that satisfaction rose during the crisis and has since fallen slightly but remains higher than prepandemic levels. During the pandemic, doctors experienced more public appreciation than they had previously, a stark contrast to what many health-care workers experienced in the US. Overall physician satisfaction was, by far, the lowest in the UK, the only place I could find with lower patient satisfaction than the US. Indeed, at the time of writing this, UK physicians have voted to take historic labor action with strikes occurring now and more planned for the weeks ahead. Low wages are a significant issue, but physicians also cite conditions for patients as a significant factor. Interestingly, issues identified in the US such as loss of autonomy and high administrative burden were far less significant in the UK.

Another measure of physician satisfaction could be emigration. According to data from the Canadian Medical Association, the number of US-trained physicians working in Canada grew less than 3% from 1996 to 2005 (up from 493 to 506) but jumped 42% from 2006 to 2014 (508 to 721). One factor could be compensation. In the US, private practice family physicians aren't paid for their services up to 30% of the time, whereas under a single-payor system, only about 2% of billings aren't covered. Moreover, dealing with insurance companies and filing claims is so bureaucratic and labor-intensive that it requires increased staff in the US compared to Canada—some estimates are as high as five times more. This eats into any profit margin a physician's office can expect to realize. However, in addition to the prospect of greater pay and fewer bureaucratic headaches, physicians are citing the opportunity to provide better care for patients as a reason for migrating north.

Another important consideration is the distribution of salaries for physicians. Traditionally, subspecialists have earned higher salaries—about 50% more than primary care doctors. With the introduction of health insurance, it became possible for many people to afford expensive surgery, and surgeons could expect to be paid for most, if not virtually all, of their cases. Beginning in the early 1900s but expanding rapidly in the 1950s and even further with Medicaid and Medicare in the 1960s, the majority of Americans could expect their hospitalization and surgeons' fees to be covered by public or private insurance. Prescription drug benefits and coverage for office visits were added later and still, to this day, tend to come with co-payments. One consequence of this dichotomy was that surgeons could earn more money than their medical counterparts. At first, this was not due to higher rates but simply that a larger proportion of surgeries were paid for, as a virtue of insurance. Office visits cost very little by comparison and were not in as dire need of an insurance safety net.

Over time, surgeries got more complex; and for some types (i.e., heart surgery, brain surgery), surgeons performing them were in greater demand. Standardization of charges as a function of coding also memorialized the relative costs of some procedures, and if technology reduced the costs, charges may not have reset. The costs of certain medical procedures, such as endoscopic procedures (those involving a scope) or catheterization (putting a catheter into a vessel to inject dye), also come from relative pricing of the surgical alternatives. All this means that doctors who perform procedures generally make more money than those who don't. So-called invasive cardiologists, those who do cardiac cauterizations, can earn two to three times the salary of their noninvasive counterparts. Justification for higher salaries also comes from more years of training that are generally required to perform procedures, but the system is clearly biased toward what a doctor does versus his/her knowledge or clinical judgment—two traits that are at least as important as technical skill.

However, over the last two or three decades, another consideration has influenced physician salaries: value to the hospital. Various business considerations can alter this value. In general, physicians who bring in patients and perform procedures that improve the hospital's bottom line are valued over physicians who do not. Indeed, physicians' salaries may bear little relationship to how much they bill.

For example, if a hospital wants a liver transplant program, it may have to pay more for a transplant surgeon than the surgeon's billing can cover. The management may decide that the value of the program to the hospital is great enough that it can cover the difference. It may take this money out of the revenue from the transplants themselves or it may pay other physicians less than is billed for on their behalf. When the hospital employs the doctors, it can dictate the rules. For example, if the medical doctors caring for the transplant patients generate ten million dollars in revenue from their physicians' services, the hospital might use eight million dollars to pay the doctors and use another million to augment the surgeons' salaries, and the remaining million might be used for "administrative overhead"—a loose term for sure. If physicians were independent, hospitals would have a harder time manipulating the system, and reimbursement for physician services would actually go into paying the physicians who provided the service to the patient rather than to the hospital.

However, the biggest redistributing of wealth among hospital-employed physicians comes from their roles in running the business. When physicians are employed by the hospital, they answer to various physicians who are in charge of whatever service line they are working in.

So for example, an emergency department has a director who has administrative responsibility for the emergency medicine doctors working there. Above the unit directors are department heads, and above them is usually a chief of staff for the hospital. In the past, these administrative positions were filled by clinicians who performed these duties alongside their clinical work. They generally received a small administrative stipend until you got to the chief of staff position where the stipend was usually more substantial. Over time, as hospital systems became more corporate in their structure, positions began to emerge within that structure that were clearly designed to bring physicians into the hospital management. Chief quality officer, chief safety officer, chief medical informatics officer, chief medical education officer, to name but a few of the myriad of management positions that have been established within large hospitals or hospital systems. Sometimes the salary that comes with these roles far exceeds the money the physician earns caring for patients. Indeed, many who serve in these roles have little or even no direct patient care responsibility. It can be confusing to understand what some of these senior positions are for and what those who hold them actually do. However, they seem to be becoming a regular fixture of modern hospital organizational charts.

An important feature of these positions is that they are created within the business leadership structure, and individuals holding these titles and receiving the salaries that go with them do so at the pleasure of senior management. These individuals often serve more traditional roles at the same time, such as a department chair. Today, it is not uncommon for a chair of medicine, for example, to also hold a position as chief medical operations officer or vice president of patient services or some other such title. What's clear is that these positions serve to cement the relationship between physician leadership and hospital business leadership. Indeed, the lines between medical practice and the business of medicine have become extremely blurred.

In his 2007 novel, Standard of Care,[2] David Kerns provides a fictional account of a well-respected internist, Dr. Daniel Fazen, who, after twenty-five years in private practice, becomes the new senior medical executive at his beloved community hospital to which he has admitted patients for years. At first, Fazen likes the job and sees his new role as guardian of quality as a natural, if easier and better-paying, extension of his years of experience as a physician. However, the hospital is soon acquired by a large multistate health-care corporation and one with a reputation as a ruthless for-profit

---

[2] David Kerns, *Standard of Care* (Sentient Publications, 2007).

hospital conglomerate. Fazen is offered big money to stay on and even convinces himself that he can do more good from within the system. Gradually, he is forced to compromise his ethics in a variety of decisions that are motivated by the interests of the hospital but that can, to some degree, be rationalized from a clinical perspective. Eventually, it crosses that line, and Dr. Fazen is forced to decide between a comfortable salary and what he believes is right. He and his wife have just purchased their dream house overlooking the San Francisco Bay, and their children are starting expensive universities. He has a lot to lose.

The novel paints a very realistic picture of the slippery slope that many physicians find themselves on when they take on business roles within a hospital organization. Many fail to grasp the important differences between an administrative role within a hospital and the role of an officer of a corporation. Some embrace the role and eagerly put on the suit, but for others, it's a gradual process, a winding road paved with reservations. For patients, it may be very confusing. That kindly doctor in the white coat coming to see them doesn't introduce himself as a business executive, yet that is exactly what he is.

However, while the chief "this or that" officer of a health system has no excuse for failing to appreciate the conflicts of interest that are inherent in his/her role, a physician who has been hired to simply be a good doctor may not immediately see the danger. Yet as we have seen with multiple examples, physicians are constantly being caught up in their employer's conflicts of interests. Not long before I started writing this book, a colleague of mine informed me that he was leaving medicine and taking a job in the pharmaceutical industry. I remember thinking to myself that he is such a good doctor, why would he want to do this? As though he could read my mind, he looked at me and said: "I just don't feel that I'm able to help patients the way I used to." He looked very sad, and suddenly, I realized what he meant.

"It's hard when the hospital ties our hands," I said.

"Not just that," he replied, "they also force our hands and hold our mouths shut."

We were in a public space that was starting to get even less private, so he stopped talking, but I knew exactly what he meant.

CHAPTER 7

Let's Compare

The harvest is always more fruitful in another man's field.

—Ovid

Before we begin to examine potential solutions to the problems facing American healthcare from employer-based conflicts of interest and hospital business models that are not aligned with patient interests, it will be illustrative to draw some comparisons between the US and other countries. At the same time, however, we should not ignore differences between different health-care systems within the US. Different systems exist, such as private and public hospital systems, the Department of Veterans' Affairs (VA) hospitals, and various health-care delivery models across different states. Comparisons between healthcare in the US and in other countries is an obvious exercise to gain insight into what we might do to reform our system or, conversely, what we might want to avoid. We can learn as much from others' failures as we can their successes. A growing number of government agencies have focused attention on this area in recent years.

Similarly, academic groups, foundations, and the press have provided their own analyses. Perhaps unsurprisingly, there is little agreement among analysts. Comparisons between many things across countries is challenging, if not impossible, at some level. Individual preferences and social context are crucial to these comparisons. Which countries have the best cuisine? Ask ten seasoned travelers, and you are likely to get ten different answers.

More surprisingly, the number of books, articles, and government reports that examine differences within the US, either across systems (e.g., veterans hospitals, public hospitals, and private hospitals) or between individual states, is quite small relative to international comparisons. This is surprising because these comparisons are much easier. There are far fewer cultural, social, and economic differences between Minnesota and Florida compared to the US and Japan. As such, analyzing differences in healthcare between states ought to be a lot easier and, at some level, more informative.

What's clear, however, is that there is an extensive body of work comparing health-care systems around the world and within the US. Entire books have been written just comparing a few countries, sometimes only superficially. Entire series have been compiled, such as those by the European Observatory and the Commonwealth Fund. In this chapter, I will not attempt to summarize this work in a comprehensive manner. Instead, I will attempt to examine the systems in other countries with an eye toward how they differ with respect to conflicts between the interests of health-care institutions, chiefly hospitals, and the interests of patients. I will compare systems along these lines by assessing the extent to which these conflicts are disclosed and managed and the extent to which interests are aligned between providers and patients. I will conduct this analysis mainly using published data, but I will supplement this with interviews of a small number of physicians working in various countries.

In the late 1990s, the World Health Organization (WHO) carried out the first ever analysis of the world's health systems. Using five performance indicators to measure health systems in 191 member states, it found that France provides the best overall healthcare among major countries, followed by Italy, Spain, Oman, Austria, and Japan. The report, published in February of 2000, has been widely criticized for its methodology, but it is just as often cited as the definitive ranking of health-care systems. The US ranked thirty-seventh.

While many of the conclusions reached by the WHO report can be criticized for their subjective nature, several objective differences can be seen between the US and other countries, and at least two of these are indisputably important—how much we pay for healthcare and life expectancy. Indeed, the most striking statistics highlighting differences in US healthcare compared to other high-income countries is that we spend the most on healthcare as a share of the economy (nearly twice as much as the average), yet we enjoy the lowest life expectancy and highest suicide rates among the eleven nations of the Organisation for Economic Co-operation and Development (OECD). While life expectancy is influenced by many factors, in a country where the majority population is descended from Europeans, it is fair to say that the genetic determinants of life span ought to be comparable. Furthermore, if healthcare isn't at least partially about improving life expectancy, what is it for?

Given these statistics, it's easy to appreciate how the Centers for Medicare and Medicaid Services (CMS) has had a relatively easy time across political parties arguing the necessity for change. A common interpretation of these statistics is that the US spends too much on unnecessary care and not enough on preventive healthcare. Although this explanation is overly simplistic, it's not without merit. US physicians order more than twice as many MRI scans per capita than their Canadian or Dutch counterparts. However, in France, the numbers are similar to the US, and they are even higher in Germany. Yet spending on healthcare as a proportion of GDP is about the same in France and Germany and 50% lower than in the US. The US performs more hip replacements per capita than almost any other OECD country, but the highest rates are in Switzerland, and their health-care spending is also far lower than ours. What's clear is that while utilization rates in the US are not always highest among various categories, we usually rank in the top three and, overall, tend to be at or near the top across the board. If utilization was like the Olympics, we would surely have a very impressive medal count indeed.

So high utilization for expensive diagnostic and therapeutic procedures such as MRIs and hip replacements may seem to support the argument that we focus too much on treatment and not enough on prevention. However, the US outperforms other similar countries in terms of various preventive measures. It has one of the highest rates of breast cancer screening among women ages fifty to sixty-nine and the second-highest rate (after the UK) of flu vaccinations among people age sixty-five and older. Thus, it's not clear that a lack of attention to preventive measures is an explanation for high costs and low life expectancy. What is clear, however, is that the US has the highest chronic disease burden and obesity rate of any OECD country. Interestingly and perhaps relatedly, Americans visit the doctor less often than citizens of most other countries, have shorter visits when they do, and have a harder time finding a physician to see at all because of a lower supply of physicians in the US than in any other OECD country.

Of course, all this utilization would be expected to result in a better cared for the populace, but this does not appear to be the case at all. At least from a life-expectancy standpoint, we finish dead last, more than two years below the OECD average and four years or more below Switzerland, Norway, France, and Australia. Black Americans have the lowest life expectancy, prompting many observers to say that health-care disparities are to blame. However, it's interesting to note that White Americans have significantly shorter life spans compared to Hispanics and Asians living in the US. It should also be noted that life expectancy also varies across the states. The top ten states by longevity all have life expectancies above eighty years and are more in line with the OECD country average. Blacks living in Hawaii actually have an average life expectancy more than seven years longer than Whites in West Virginia.

Similarly, if we examine the way health-care systems are set up across countries, we find some pretty stark differences. Although T. R. Reid's *New York Times'* bestseller *Healing of America: A Global Quest for Better, Cheaper, and Fairer Health Care*[1] is now more than a decade old, his depiction of healthcare in the US compared to France, Germany, Japan, the United Kingdom, and Canada is still relevant. Although the characterizations provided are simplistic, the basic "models" described by Reid are useful as a starting point. Reid,

---

[1] T. R. Reid, *Healing of America: A Global Quest for Better, Cheaper, and Fairer Health Care* (Penguin Press, 2010).

who refers to the US as having a health-care market rather than a system, describes four major models for healthcare.

The *Beveridge Model* was adopted by Britain and is closest to socialized medicine, according to Reid. Here almost all health-care providers work as government employees, the government acts as the single-payor for all health services, and patients incur no out-of-pocket costs. The *Bismarck Model*, also known as the Social Health Insurance Model, began in Germany under Otto von Bismarck. Although the system today has undergone many changes to the one first introduced in 1883, it is still based on payment of fees into a fund that, in turn, pays health-care providers, which can be government-owned or private institutions. The insurance coverage is also mainly provided through private companies. However, the insurance companies operate as nonprofits and are required to sign up all citizens without any conditions. The government plays a central role in determining payments for various health services, thus exercising some control on cost. The *National Health Insurance Model*, such as in Canada and Norway, has a single-payor system like Britain; however, the health-care providers work mostly as private entities. Finally, the *Out-of-Pocket Model* is followed in most poor countries. There is no public or private system of health insurance. People mostly pay for the services they receive out of pocket. However, this leaves many underprivileged people without essential healthcare. Almost all countries with such a system have a much lower life expectancy and high infant mortality rates.

Reid describes the health-care system in the US as following many of the international systems in bits and pieces. For most working people under sixty-five, the Bismarck Model adopted by Germany and Japan is the closest. However, in America, health insurance companies can be for-profit enterprises unlike in Germany and Japan, and many of the issues raised by critics of insurance companies in the US are not applicable in these other countries. The model for Native Americans, military personnel, and veterans is like the Beveridge Model of Britain, where the government acts as both the payor and provider. For those over sixty-five, the US uses a model very close to the Canadian single-payor model. The government ends up acting as the insurer while the private sector provides the medical services. Finally, for uninsured Americans, the model ends up looking like the out-of-pocket model used in various underdeveloped countries. Most of the medical facilities are too expensive for these people, and they are left with virtually no healthcare. As we'll see, this is a reasonable summary of the US system, but it's actually even more complex.

In an interesting twist, Reid attempts to get treatment for a shoulder condition in various countries and documents his experiences in the book. In the UK, he is told by a British doctor to live with his shoulder problem, that the system would not treat it, and that every other British doctor would tell him the same thing. In Canada, Reid could obtain surgical care at a reasonable cost, but he would have to wait eighteen months to receive it. He also finds suitable treatment in India, which has an out-of-pocket model, the only one Reid considers to be worse than the American system of healthcare.

Various other authors have examined how healthcare differs around the word. A comprehensive textbook entitled *Comparative Health Systems: A Global Perspective* by James A. Johnson, PhD, MPA,

MSc; Carleen Stoskopf, ScD; and Leiyu Shi, DrPH, MBA, MPA[2] is in its second edition, published in 2018. Even more recently, Ezekiel (Zeke) Emanuel, MD, notable oncologist and bioethicist, tries to answer the question "Which country has the world's best healthcare?" in a book with this title published in 2020.[3] Spoiler alert, he doesn't actually tell us. Instead, Emanuel provides a scholarly, if somewhat dry, examination of the advantages and disadvantages of each system and hints at some of the ways these systems have addressed similar problems. Some of their solutions have also produced different problems, echoing many of our own. Emanuel notes that Germany, the Netherlands, Norway, and, rather curiously, Taiwan are among the best-performing when twenty-two different criteria are considered. The US is near the bottom.

Emanuel argues that healthcare is "path-dependent," meaning that the effects of preexisting institutional structures determine what new structures can look like. He reviews the history of healthcare in each of the eleven countries he focuses on and tries to explain how these histories interact with culture and population preferences to land us where we are. Emanuel dispels many myths about healthcare in other countries and helps explain why these myths are popular with politicians from both ends of the political spectrum.

Canada, for example, is held up by some as a sterling example of a sensible one-payor system, while to others, it's a perfect example of the perils of socialized medicine. In truth, there is no single

---

[2] James A. Johnson, PhD, MPA, MSc; Carleen Stoskopf, ScD; and Leiyu Shi, DrPH, MBA, MPA, *Comparative Health Systems: A Global Perspective, Second Edition* (Jones & Bartlett, 2018).

[3] Ezekiel "Zeke" Emanuel, MD, *Which Country has the World's Best Healthcare?* (Public Affairs Press, 2020).

Canadian system. Although they share common principles, there are thirteen different provincial and territorial health-care systems, some of which are more different from one another than they are from systems in other countries entirely. However, across Canada, there is universal medical coverage for all its citizens with no co-payments for hospitalization, diagnostic tests, or physician visits. There is no universal prescription drug coverage, however, no long-term care coverage, and services such as ambulances, dental, and vision are not uniformly covered by the thirteen systems. Despite being branded as socialized medicine by its detractors, healthcare delivery in Canada is almost exclusively provided through nongovernmental institutions. Patients can choose their physicians and have free access to specialists. Although wait times for elective procedures are often overblown by conservative commentators, long wait times do exist at many Canadian hospitals and may be related to the lack of activity-based payment systems.

By contrast, the National Health Service (NHS) in the United Kingdom is truly a socialized system with healthcare financed through the use of general income tax revenues and the delivery system almost exclusively government-controlled. A small private system runs in parallel to the NHS, but it is not integral to the system. This is unlike similar systems in France and Australia where the public systems encourage and rely on functioning private insurance markets. The NHS is perhaps the most studied health-care system in the world. One measure of its success, perhaps the most important, is that it remains very popular with the citizens it serves. Yet the NHS has struggled with physician and nursing shortages, deteriorating conditions of many of its hospitals, and slow adoption of new technologies, including new drugs, devices, and electronic health records. The UK has fewer hospital beds and a longer average length of stay compared to the US leading to high hospital occupancy rates. This situation was particularly perilous during the COVID-19 pandemic, and there was no capacity to deal with the surge in demand. Relatedly, wait times for elective procedures, physician appointments, and even cancer care tend to be long and continue to be a major challenge for the system and a sore point for both patients and providers. Given that the UK spends less on healthcare as a function of GDP (9.6%) than most other OECD countries, some analysts observe that it's getting what it pays for. Efforts to improve quality of care in the NHS, such as the Quality and Outcomes Framework (QOF), have been plagued by technical and procedural problems and widely criticized as doing little to improve outcomes while being cumbersome to administer. Interestingly, while both the US and the UK are facing a long-term care crisis, the issue is barely on the political radar in the US while it was a major issue in the UK during the 2017 election.

France has a compulsory public insurance system, but its coverage is so sparse that supplemental private insurance to cover high out-of-pocket costs is essential for most people. Although there is central financing and strong national regulation, its health-care delivery systems are mostly private. The French can access any physician, including specialists, but the system is notoriously fragmented and inefficient. These limitations have fueled criticism for the WHO rankings, even among French academics. Germany offers similar, if not greater, patient choice than France, with, if you will pardon the stereotype, German efficiency. Access to physicians and hospitals is convenient. On average, Germans have a primary care physician within fifteen minutes of where they live. However, insurance, called sickness funds, are anything but efficient, with over one hundred to choose from and no apparent reason for that number since about 99% of coverage is the same across funds. Even stranger, the funds collectively bargain with hospitals to set prices—there are no individual pricing arrangements or networks. The Germans also use a single-payor system funded by taxes but rely on multiple private insurance companies to actually pay for care. Germany also has too many hospitals and hospital beds and continues to hospitalize patients for conditions that require only outpatient care most everywhere else. However, critically, Germany is one of the very few countries that has universal long-term care coverage though it only covers about 50% of the costs.

The Netherlands has similarities to the German system but with an even more comprehensive long-term care system funded by mandatory taxation. However, the Dutch system has some significant differences to other systems in Europe. The long traditions of conservative, low interventional care on the front lines delivered by general practitioners is a relatively unique aspect. These general practitioners also serve as gatekeepers who control access to specialists and generally manage and coordinate care. This "front line" is supported by a state-of-the-art system of hospitals and hospital-based specialists. Although the Dutch system wins praises from the *Eurohealth* consumer index and other groups, it's not without its flaws and contradictions. The system is essentially one of managed competition operating within a municipal framework based on cooperation. Managed competition requires selective contracting and closed networks and essentially rules out cooperation. As a result, it has not reached any significant threshold. The Dutch system is therefore extremely complex, and much of the complexity serves to undermine efficiency. At the other end of the complexity spectrum is Norway. Norway may have the least complicated/most efficient system in the world although supplemental insurance exists here too as in the Netherlands. Norway also has universal healthcare financed using a model similar to Canada and uses general practitioners to manage care and restrict access to specialists. A major problem with Norway's system is wait times for non-life-threatening specialist care, and their supplemental insurance system has grown to address this precise issue, leading to complaints over access inequity. Norway also has no funding system for long-term care, leaving patients with this burden.

Finally, rounding out the European countries on Emanuel's list is Switzerland, which does not have a single payor. The Swiss system is very popular with its citizens who may choose any doctor or hospital, do not have any appreciable wait times, and have the general impression that quality is high. Unfortunately, although it does provide universal care through insurance mandates and is held up by some as an example of successfully managed competition, costs are high and rising sharply. One measure, prescription drug costs, are the highest in the world after the US. The Swiss system is also complex and appears relatively resistant to change.

Similar to the conclusions reached by T. R. Reid, Ezekiel Emanuel concludes that the US system is an amalgamation of systems around the world. We have our own fully socialized healthcare systems administered by three separate programs: the VA for veterans, TRICARE for active-duty military, and the Indian Health Service for Native Americans. In total, these programs cover nearly thirteen million Americans or just under 4% of the population. Meanwhile, traditional Medicare Part A (hospitals) and Part B (physician services) used by 38.7 million (11.7%), as well as the Medicaid system, including the Children's Health Insurance Program (CHIP), used by an additional 89.4 million (27%), closely resemble the systems in Canada and Norway. Furthermore, like in France, Medicare recipients can buy private supplementary insurance (Medigap plans) to cover additional services not included in traditional Medicare. Finally, Medicare Advantage, used by 26.9 million (8.1%), introduced a German model where the government uses tax dollars to pay private insurance companies to administer the programs that patients select. The federally subsidized insurance exchange system with an individual insurance mandate under the Affordable Care Act is essentially the Swiss model, which currently covers 16.3 million or just under 5% of Americans. Meanwhile, traditional employer-based healthcare covers about half the population and is also subsidized through tax exclusions on these benefits. Importantly, even though about two-thirds of the population has private insurance, only a third of patients in the hospital in 2018, according to the American Hospital Association, had private insurance. Thus, while the public system "covers" only about a third of Americans, it actually pays for two-thirds of hospital bills. Finally, for uninsured Americans (as of 2023, about 8%), the model is indeed an out-of-pocket model used in various underdeveloped countries. If you noticed that these number add up to more than 100%, it's because some people have multiple sources of coverage at the same time. Emanuel describes the financing of healthcare in the US as "an incomprehensible mess that has grown up over time, devoid of design or rationality and now justification."

Thus, while comparisons across national systems can be informative, the complexity that exists when looking at each system as a whole makes it challenging to examine specific aspects in isolation. Emanuel does discuss alignment of health systems to the goals of patients, but the potential for conflicts of interest between the interests of hospitals and of patients is not discussed.

Even with the Affordable Care Act of 2010, roughly 8% of Americans are uninsured while nearly everyone is covered by a healthcare system in most other high-income countries. Furthermore, the types of insurance that patients have can determine their access to care or willingness to pay for preventive healthcare even when they know it's in their best interest. As a result, rates of preventable hospitalizations for diseases like diabetes and hypertension are much lower in countries like Canada and Switzerland compared to the US though rates are even higher than the US in Germany, the only high-income country with higher rates than the US. However, this is at least in part related to Germans' willingness to admit patients to the hospital to "get their disease under control," a practice that largely disappeared in the US a generation ago. So, for example, a newly diagnosed diabetic or hypertensive might actually be admitted to the hospital to get them on a stable treatment regimen, something that is now unheard of in even small-town community hospitals in America.

However, how do various countries differ with respect to the main factors considered in this book, namely, employer-based conflict of interest, hospital business models and funding, regulation, and physician and patient satisfaction? Well, for starters, in countries that have a form of socialized medicine, employer-based conflicts of interest are neither as common nor as gratuitous. However, they can still exist. Cost cutting is still a fact of daily life for hospitals everywhere. Interestingly, health-care spending in proportion to GDP is increasing in all OECD member countries. Furthermore, the rate of increase in spending over the last decade is actually quite similar to the US, if even slightly higher. It's just that we had such runaway health-care spending in the 1980s and 1990s that we entered the twenty-first century at levels other countries are only reaching now. So, with costs rising, societies all over the planet are seeking to spend less, and although the moral grounds may be less dubious, a hospital or national health system that chooses to restrict the use of some technology or medication because it's too expensive does enter into a conflict of interest between society's interest in spending less and a patient's acute interest in having something better. Do physicians in other countries find themselves in the middle of this conflict the way they do in the US?

Interestingly, most other OECD countries have been implementing some form of value-based healthcare for some time now. An important difference, though, is that with a more socialized health-care system, any savings is returned to the public rather than to a cabal of executives and shareholders. It's also, by design, more transparent. When societies have to pay higher taxes to get more or better healthcare, they can directly ask what they are getting; and if they choose to cut costs, they can examine whether the cuts removed access to things most people want. By contrast, the US system is murky and secretive. If costs can be cut, there is no mechanism to return the savings to the public, and there is vast incentive to enrich the very people making the decisions. A more striking and obvious conflict of interest would be hard to imagine.

What do doctors working in these various countries think about these issues? I asked this question to dozens of doctors working in different countries around the world. I was surprised by some of their answers while other answers were rather predictable. For example, I was not surprised to learn that most doctors in every country feel a decrease in satisfaction compared to ten years ago. The reasons varied, but there is a general sense among physicians that medicine is becoming less rewarding. The COVID-19 pandemic was clearly a factor, but for most countries, physician satisfaction was in decline even before COVID-19. Administrative burden, pay, and reduced autonomy were common themes regardless of the relative starting point for individual countries. Interestingly, physician "wellness" programs don't exist in most countries, but where they do, doctors I spoke to tended to see them as teaching coping skills rather than addressing underlying problems affecting physician satisfaction.

I was surprised to learn how, in many countries, budgets are set at the hospital or department level, and these budgets serve to cap spending in peculiar ways. For example, one Dutch physician explained that in the Netherlands, when the annual budget for abdominal surgery is used up, hospitals stop elective surgery and focus only on emergencies. This obviously causes hardship for patients who need to wait, but it is obviously very inefficient as well. Most of the costs associated with maintaining an abdominal surgery program are fixed. Physicians and nurses are still being paid. Just as strangely, in the UK, each hospital or hospital system has a budget, but labor costs are set at the national level. I was also surprised to learn that in many systems, budgets were often exceeded, and the only effect was for governmental agencies to examine the problem, usually concluding that the problem could not be avoided for that budget cycle and then injecting public funds to shore up the system. Conversely, budget surpluses were often used to buy new equipment or for other nonrecurring spending. Few systems use pay for performance, and the few that do are largely seen as ineffective. No doctors outside the US admitted to any form of financial incentives, direct or indirect for themselves, based on containing hospital costs.

Of the physicians I spoke with, Japanese doctors seemed to enjoy the greatest professional autonomy among their colleagues in other high-income countries, certainly much greater than most physicians in the US. However, even in Japan, doctors working in hospitals have to work within budgetary constraints, and although they are, in theory, free to practice as they see fit, there are professional norms that indirectly limit their practices. This is similar to what physicians in the UK and in Belgium told me. Dutch physicians told me that while they enjoy considerable professional autonomy, a strong tradition of conservative care still motivates practice in the Netherlands. Even in very interventionist settings like the ICU, Dutch physicians feel they are less aggressive with therapies than many other Europeans.

With respect to adoption of innovation, most physicians told me that their system had structures, some quite cumbersome, to determine if new drugs and devices would be made available. In essence, most countries, like the US, use their regulatory agencies to determine safety and efficacy, but cost-effectiveness was left to the health-care system to determine. In the UK, there is a national organization that evaluates new technologies and makes recommendations, but individual hospitals are free to make their own decisions. Thus, even in countries with a single national system, there can be variation in the decision to adopt a technology at the local or regional level. This appears to be true in our own VA system as some VA hospitals offer treatments that others do not. Conversely, in some countries that use a patchwork of insurance companies, for example, in Germany where there are more than one hundred, variation in treatments offered is no greater, and it may even be less.

Thus, the pictures painted by physicians working in various other countries reinforce many of the observations made by Reid, Emanuel, and others studying this area. However, while we may be able to learn from the advances and mistakes of other countries, when it comes to corporate healthcare and employer-based conflicts of interest, we are largely out on our own. The medical-industrial complex of the United States is unique among high-income countries.

Importantly, few authors have critically examined the rather striking differences in healthcare within the US. Yes, the delivery of healthcare in the US differs, sometimes dramatically, from other high-income countries, but there are also important differences *within* the US. Different systems exist such as private and public hospital systems, the VA hospitals, and various health-care delivery models across different states. For example, if we isolate the state of California, the fifth largest economy in the world, we find life expectancies above the OECD country average; and in 2014, the last year compiled by CMS, health-care spending per capita was $7,549, lower than thirty-six other states. Expressed as a proportion of GDP for that year, California health-care spending was only 10.8%, compared to 17.1% for the US as a whole, and in line with many OECD countries. Meanwhile, Massachusetts is notable for being the state that has come closest to universal coverage with more than 98% of its citizens insured under its implementation of the Affordable Care Act. Massachusetts also established a health policy commission in 2012 to define a limit on health-care cost growth based on state GDP and the mean age of the population. Similarly, in 2014, Maryland enacted legislation that limits increases in per capita hospital spending to historical averages. Other states have adopted or are looking to adopt similar approaches. Maryland is also unique among states for its all-payor rate-setting policy. In other states, Medicare pays one rate for each diagnostic category or diagnosis-related group (DRG). Medicaid pays another, typically lower rate, and individual private insurance companies negotiate rates individually with each hospital system, typically arriving at a multiple (i.e., one and half, two times, etc.) of the Medicare rate. However, in Maryland, since the 1970s, an independent commission determines the rates for each DRG regardless of who is paying, Medicare, Medicaid, or private insurance. This practice is similar to France, the Netherlands, and Germany and has resulted in below average health-care cost increases for the state over time. Thus, individual states serve as useful comparisons that are far easier and with less baggage than international comparisons.

A final place to look for comparisons is between the VA System, our own socialized medicine system, and the rest of the health-care system. Interestingly, many of the problems plaguing socialized systems in other countries were in full display here as well. Not long ago, the Department of Veterans Affairs health-care system was a dysfunctional, scandal-prone bureaucracy. Quality was poor, and wait times for care were long. However, as Phillip Longman writes in *Best Care Anywhere: Why VA Health Care Is Better Than Yours*, the system has been transformed into the benchmark for high-quality medicine in the US. Longman argues that much of what we think we know about health, healthcare, and medical economics are just plain wrong. The VA system is now extraordinarily cost-effective and has proven to be highly popular with veterans. Longman goes on to make the case for how both Medicare and private insurance have failed to address many of the problems facing US healthcare and have reinforced the need for applying the lessons of the VA.

When I spoke with doctors working in the VA system, including those who have also worked in the private sector, they confirm that VA care is high-quality and that many of the traditional complaints of the VA such as long delays for access have been substantially improved. However, VA physicians express skepticism that a VA-style health-care system could work for most Americans. One physician told me that veterans are used to "not having things" and that the VA is very good about getting you what you need but not necessarily everything you may want. Physicians that I spoke to working in the VA system are highly supportive of its goals and structure. They believe the system provides good care, and although they are aware of constraints on what they can prescribe, as well as gaps between what they can offer patients and what they may want, they express the view that the system has processes and that they are equitable. However, the system is still quite bureaucratic and slow to change. If these sentiments sound similar to the NHS in the UK, it's probably not a coincidence. The British are rather notorious for their "stiff upper lip" mentality, and many view certain types of medical care considered standard in the US as luxuries. Perhaps unsurprisingly and Longman's claims notwithstanding, there is little call for an NHS or VA-style system for all Americans. Calls for a single-payor system are more likely about extending Medicare for all, moving us toward a more Canadian or Norwegian system, perhaps with the French-styled Medicare Advantage option.

However, in the last several years, we have not sailed in either of these directions. Instead, we have drifted off course entirely. As we look at the direction healthcare in the US is heading and we look at other countries, it's clear that we are sailing into uncharted waters. No system in the world has a corporate system of healthcare where large corporations control not just hospitals and insurance providers but also the professionals who work in these institutions. Never before have we had a majority of doctors in this country employed by corporations, and if current trends are any indication, the transformation to an exclusively corporate system is just around the corner. Even where state laws prohibit hospitals from directly employing physicians, workarounds such as the Permanente Medical Groups in California, which use mutually exclusive contracts with the two other branches of the Kaiser system (Kaiser Foundation Health Plans and Kaiser Foundation Hospitals), nevertheless, create a *de facto* corporate system.

As I have illustrated using both published evidence and first-hand accounts, doctors around the world face important challenges to providing high-quality care to patients. Rising costs and the ever-increasing complexity of medicine are common themes, but each country faces unique challenges. While physicians in several but not all other countries experience conflict between the demands of the system and the needs of patients, none experience this more than US physicians. No other health-care system in the world has combined a health insurance company, a hospital network, and all physicians caring for patients interacting with these entities under one private organization. Most physicians I have spoken to in other countries express surprise that such a system with such obvious inherent conflicts of interest could be allowed to exist, much less allowed to become a dominant model.

Good Medicine or Good Business?

Wisdom considers not only the cost of a choice but also its value.

—Wes Fesler

At the heart of value-based healthcare is the assessment of value. What something costs is definable, trackable, and can even be negotiated. What something is worth is another matter.

Beginning in the 1980s, a system known as evidence-based medicine (EBM) was introduced to make the practice of medicine more scientific and accountable. EBM is not only about cost. It is a system to judge whether one therapy should be used over another. Indeed, cost may not even factor in or may be only a minor consideration. One output of EBM research is to express benefit or lack of benefit from a certain therapy in terms of the number (of patients) needed to treat (NNT) to achieve the desired outcome. The larger this number is, the smaller is the effect of the intervention—in other words, when more patients need to be treated to achieve one positive outcome. Similarly, researchers can examine harm attributable to the therapy, such as adverse effects, and can calculate a NNH (number needed to harm). The NNT may be weighted differently than the NNH because the potential benefit may be great and the potential harms only slight. Conversely, the benefit could be relatively small, but the harm could be great (i.e., death). Under these circumstances, the difference between NNT and NNH would have to be very large.

A drug to reduce hair loss, for example, could have a very low NNT—only a few patients would need to be treated to achieve a success. Indeed, a perfect NNT is 1, and such a drug would be effective 100% of the time. However, if the drug had a fatal side effect, the effect would have to be extremely rare and, thus, equate to a very large NNH. You might wonder how we would ever accept a treatment that had a potential for death if the benefit was only cosmetic. In fact, there are many examples of therapies or products in general that have some risk, yet we use them even though the benefit is small or even debatable. Cosmetics themselves frequently cause allergic reactions, and while most are mild, fatalities have occurred. The risk is so small, however, that most consumers are willing to take it. A similar example concerns Botox injections. Botox is derived from botulinum toxin and could prove fatal if injected intravenously in sufficient quantities. Estimates of fatal reactions to Botox, however, are very low. Just sixteen deaths were reported between 1997 and 2006. Given that about three million Botox injects are performed each year, the risk of death would be about one in two million. This puts it on par with the risk of getting a COVID-19 vaccine or driving about one hundred miles.

While costs may not be a consideration when evaluating therapies, quite often, costs do become a consideration, and NNT is a convenient, perhaps too convenient, way to express aggregate cost to benefit. If, for example, the NNT for a drug is one hundred and the therapy costs ten thousand dollars, we can safely conclude that it will cost one million dollars to achieve a single positive outcome. Even if the outcome is survival, society will likely reject this therapy. This analysis also allows drug and biomedical device manufacturers to set prices. If the treatment was only ten dollars, the cost of one life saved would only be one thousand dollars. However, this alone would not ensure its acceptance. With an NNT of one hundred, the safety profile would have to be extremely good. If the risk of serious adverse events was high, say 20% (or an NNH of five) for something dreadful and irreversible like blindness, the drug would never be approved, much less prescribed, regardless of the cost.

Of course, not all outcomes are as obviously beneficial as survival, and even survival deserves some qualification. A therapy for stroke that improves your chances to survive but not return to normal function is obviously less valuable than one that returns you to your prior state.

Beginning in the 1960s, researchers introduced a concept that would revolutionize value assessment and not just in medicine. A quality-adjusted life year or QALY is an estimate of how much a particular treatment or product will not just increase your life span but also do so in relation to quality of life. Researchers with training in what is known as cost-effectiveness analysis use various methods (some controversial) to determine how many QALYs something can achieve and factor in both the NNT to achieve it along with NNH.

Societies, for their parts, can then set specific thresholds to determine if something is worth the cost by expressing the cost per QALY.

Driver's side airbags are said to cost twenty-four thousand dollars per QALY (in 1993 dollars), an amount widely deemed reasonable by US sensibilities at the time. Dual front-seat airbags, on the other hand, increase the cost to sixty-one thousand dollars per QALY, leading some to argue that they are not cost-effective. Nevertheless, they have become mandatory on all new cars.

From a societal perspective, there is a great need to put healthcare in a cost-effectiveness framework. When interventions are very expensive or even when they are only moderately expensive but are very common such that the total costs become significant, society has the right to ask, "Is this the best way to use limited resources?"

The problem is that formal cost-effectiveness analyses can be complicated to perform on many medical or surgical treatments, and experts don't agree on all the various inputs and the assumptions underlying them. As a result, there is no master catalogue to look up the cost-effectiveness of each therapy and make an objective assessment as to whether it is above or below the threshold. When the analysis is more straightforward, say for a new cancer drug, the threshold usually used is fifty thousand dollars to one hundred thousand dollars per QALY. When an agreed-upon cost per QALY is not available, which is the norm, physicians and hospital administrators are free to use their judgment. Unfortunately, for reasons enumerated already, they tend to be stingy—particularly if there are cheaper alternatives that work almost as well. If the cost of a new therapy is high but there are no treatment alternatives, most hospitals will acquiesce.

However, if a new therapy has certain advantages over existing thera-pies, it's a judgment call as to how much those advantages are worth.

For example, two hypothetical anesthetics have similar safety profiles, but the older drug has the disadvantage of coming off slowly and leaving patients groggy and nauseated for as long as twenty-four hours. Seeing these features as undesirable, a drug company spends several years and several million dollars to develop a new drug, which comes off quickly and leaves patients refreshed and not nauseous. No one disagrees that the newer drug is better, but the drug company charges five times the cost of the old drug. The result is an extra five hundred dollars per surgery. Even if a formal cost-effectiveness analy-sis could be done, the QALYs the new drug provides are close to zero per case because twenty-four hours of feeling better doesn't materially affect your overall quality of life. So the cost per QALY would be astronomical. In a true value-based model, however, patients would have a say as to whether they value the drug sufficiently for this cost; and if they do, the costs might well be passed along to the consumer as per the rest of the free market economy. However, in healthcare, the equation is different. The hospital looks at how many surgeries it does per year, let's say twenty thousand, and determines that use of this new drug will cost the hospital ten million dollars a year. Under the current system and under every value-based model yet proposed, hospitals are in conflict between their own financial well-being and their desire to do something better for patients. When decisions like this are made at the systems level, it's easy to make them impersonal; and when prevailing attitudes are distorted by the *big lie* in health-care, it's easy to decide that a bit of temporary unpleasantness just isn't worth ten million dollars, even for twenty thousand sick, helpless individuals who have no say in the matter. When you then place what amounts to a bounty on this decision by tying cost reductions to administrator bonuses, you make the conflict of interest very personal with the decision-maker, and the outcome is almost assured.

Of course, this problem is not unique to US healthcare. If the National Health Service of the UK was confronted with the same scenario, its administrators would be confronted with the same trade-offs, only at a larger scale. The NHS performs about ten million surgeries a year, so spending an extra five hundred dollars on each would drive up the costs by five billion dollars! Of course, it might be a political win to spend this money and avail the public of a true benefit. Further, these decisions are never so simple. At a systems level, the NHS could negotiate the cost of the new drug and perhaps only pay three hundred dollars, leading to a smaller increase of three billion dollars per year. Across the entire NHS, the use of a drug that allows patients to recover faster from surgery could change patient throughput sufficiently to save money in other ways, including time in hospital, staffing, etc. In the end, the drug could even result in a net saving. However, only if it were actually adopted would we be able to determine its impact, which it might never be if the five-billion-dollar price tag was seen as a nonstarter.

The free market system in US healthcare might also have a role to play in these kinds of decisions. If hospital A decided not to adopt the new drug because it didn't want to spend the ten million dollars, hospital B might decide to adopt it as competitive advantage. Hospital B might reason that it might steal away a portion of hospital A's business by offering the treatment and might estimate that the ten million dollars it spends will be more than offset by the additional business it gains. Hospital B might even be able to strike a deal with the drug manufacturer so its costs are reduced, at least for a time, since the company will know that, eventually, hospital A will have to adopt the therapy to compete. These effects of competition are touted as advantages of a free market system. The problem with our health-care system is that it's not a free market. For one thing, insurance providers generally determine which hospital a patient can use, not the patient themselves. Furthermore, so-called value-based payment plans won't fix this problem because, at the end of day, they are really about holding down costs; and as we can see in this example, some things of value will unavoidably increase costs.

Unfortunately, these examples paint a picture that is decidedly more logical than the system actually is. Evidence-based medicine has inadvertently given rise to the physician as hospital fiduciary. Hospital-employed physicians are reminded constantly that health-care is too expensive, and every effort should be made to reduce costs. The *big lie* in healthcare is usually invoked, but even when it's not, hospital employees are conditioned to think as if a single pool of money exists to pay for care and their salaries. In the extreme, this can lead to a perception that the physician is spending his or her own money on care for the patient. The temptation is far too great for the doctors to substitute their own values for their patients' when it comes to making decisions that involve cost. In this context, therapies that cost only slightly more are often seen as frivolous unless they dramatically impact outcomes. In our hypothetical anesthetic example, a physician might feel compassion for a patient who is groggy and nauseous after surgery but feel he or she would be financially irresponsible to order a therapy that would increase the costs when these conditions are not life-threatening or even long-lasting.

Even when differences in survival are demonstrated, physicians can reach seemingly bizarre conclusions. When results are pooled from several large studies evaluating survival that is achieved when various types of intravenous fluids are used, a *decrease* in survival is seen with saline, a salt solution that has been a standard of care for more than a century. The comparator fluids include various components that are commonly used in foods and other products that are used to achieve a fluid whose composition is more like blood plasma and hence thought to be more "physiologic," which is just a way of saying that it's less alien to the body. Veterinarians have long since stopped using saline for most of their patients. However, the reaction of physicians to this news, even though it's been evolving for more than a decade, has been more measured. Some have openly wondered whether a 1% survival difference is "clinically relevant" while others have noted that saline remains cheap, about one dollar for a one-liter bag, less than half the price of more modern solutions. If one looks at this from a cost-effectiveness perspective, then the NNT (number needed to treat to save one life) is 100, and the costs would be equal to about two dollars multiplied by the number of liters prescribed. Let's assume the number of liters is five, so for one thousand dollars, we can save one life. Even if we were talking about patients with advanced chronic disease whose life expectancy was only one year and even if we discounted the QALY by 50% because such patients' quality of life would not be perfect, we would still calculate a cost per QALY of only two thousand dollars. This makes eliminating saline thirty times more cost-effective than mandating front-seat airbags.

As of early 2024, the FDA has issued no guidance for the elimination of saline.

From a patient perspective, it seems quite likely that a group of one hundred would agree that spending just one thousand dollars total on the entire group (ten dollars per person) would be worth it if one more of them could leave the hospital alive. Interestingly, another solution also found to work better than saline, known as lactated Ringer's solution, costs about the same as saline, so there's not even a cost argument. Yet physicians still use saline in at least 50% of their patients. One reason for this might be that physicians don't actually know what most things cost. That's right. The very people who are making decisions about the value of various treatments not only don't know how to judge value but they also don't even know what most things cost. Physicians can be forgiven to a degree because the cost of most things in the hospital, from drugs to lab tests to supplies, are not easy to determine and can vary widely from time to time. If you type "cost of normal saline" into Google, you can see that it's offered by various suppliers for prices ranging from five dollars to two hundred dollars per liter, yet hospitals pay about one to two dollars per liter. Hospital Pharmacy and Therapeutics committees should do a better job, but even here, physician attitudes—questioning whether 1% survival difference is clinically relevant—can bias their decision-making.

As a clinician-scientist, I studied this question for many years; and for most of this time, the only evidence we had was from observational studies—analyzing data from large groups of patients and using analytic techniques to attempt to control for bias. Bias is a major concern in this kind of research because intravenous fluids were not allocated randomly to patients. A few doctors like me were sufficiently concerned about the risks of saline to prescribe other fluids to our patients, but most, indeed more than 90% of physicians, were just not convinced. A few doctors used alternative fluids only in select patients, further contributing to a potential bias in any dataset we could analyze. Working with other investigators, like Andy Shaw, MD, now at the Cleveland Clinic, we began to show in very large groups of patients from national datasets that saline was *associated* with harm. I emphasize this is only an association because observational studies can't prove a causal relationship. It's always possible that other factors, perhaps even factors we have no idea about, could be responsible for this relationship, and the fluid type was only a coincidence.

For example, maybe doctors who use alternative fluids are just better, smarter, and more capable than doctors who prescribe saline. In this way, fluid type is just a marker of something else (e.g., better doctors) that likely influences the outcome of interest: survival. As someone who prescribes alternative fluids, I'd be happy to entertain this possibility, but I don't believe it's at all likely. Still, there could be any number of alternative explanations, and this is the problem with all association studies. The fact that there were several studies like this and they included huge numbers of patients (from several thousand to more than a million) from different institutions and in different patient groups made the risk of bias lower but didn't eliminate it completely. Only a randomized trial where patients receive one type or another fluid based on an unbiased function, the equivalent of a coin toss, can truly establish a causal relationship. We did have some randomized data from small groups of patients, but it literally takes thousands to show the kinds of differences we were concerned with.

By way of example, to show that mortality can be reduced from 10% to 9%, a 1% absolute or 10% relative difference, we would need approximately twenty-six thousand patients. At the time we were doing these studies, no one had ever done a trial in the ICU of this size. We also had data from animal experiments where the underlying mortality rate was much higher and the exposure to saline much greater, and these studies did show significant differences. Perhaps this is why veterinarians were easier to convince while most physicians were still skeptical. Given that saline was an international standard, it was very hard to convince most doctors that they should use something else when the evidence we had was perceived as weak. I discussed this problem with officials at the National Institutes of Health (NIH), but the general consensus was that it would be very difficult to do a large enough study to show an effect, and it just wasn't seen as a large enough priority.

To make matters worse, comparing one drug to another is typically viewed as the sort of study a drug manufacturer would pay for as opposed to the NIH. In 2012, I took a meeting with an executive from one of the leading suppliers of an alternative, so-called balanced, intravenous fluid. I wanted to see if the company might be interested in funding a large clinical trial. After all, if the alternative fluid was shown to be safer, as I believed it was, the company ought to be able to increase its sales. However, the problem was explained to me as follows:

The company made saline, and the same company made alternatives to saline. Although the main alternative fluid the company manufactured cost about twice the price of saline, it also cost nearly twice as much to make so margins on these two products, the difference between what something cost to make and what you can sell it for, were almost the same. The executive told me that if all intravenous fluids were converted to this alternative to saline, they would make about as much money as they currently make on saline. In other words, there was no financial incentive to pay for a large clinical trial. The executive further explained to me the financial landscape was actually negative for the company because it would cost money to convert production, and because it would take a while to do so, they'd have to start making the change before the surge in demand. This would be okay as long as they got it right, and physicians, indeed, converted to the new fluid, but if they got it wrong, they'd lose money. In other words, the executive was telling me that if they changed their manufacturing plants from making saline to making this alternative fluid and physicians didn't order it, they'd lose market share to another company making saline. Conversely, if they didn't switch over, they could lose market share to a company making an alternative to saline if the demand increased more or faster than they projected. So, for the company, the status quo was best for business. The executive acknowledged that the company would do whatever was safest for patients, even if they had to pay the costs, but finding additional money to study the problem was just not going to be in the cards.

So it looked like the controversy was going to continue. Right around this time, a friend sent me a paper from the *Journal of the American Medical Association* entitled "The Abuse of Normal Salt Solution" in which the author, Dr. George H. Evevans, attempts to warn readers "against the thoughtless and indiscriminate use of [saline]."[1] The paper was published in 1911. This paper paired well with another one I'd collected from 1902 entitled "Concerning the Poisonous Effect of Pure Sodium Chloride Solutions upon the Nerve Muscle Preparation" by none other than Harvey Cushing for whom Cushing's disease, a condition in which a benign tumor in the pituitary gland signals the adrenal glands to make too much cortisol, is named. I was beginning to wonder if physicians in the twenty-third century would still be wrestling with this. However, in 2018, all this changed. Investigators from Vanderbilt University including my collaborator, Dr. Andy Shaw, mentioned above, conducted two randomized trials, one for critically ill patients going to the ICU and the other for less severe patients admitted to general floors. Collectively, the two studies enrolled nearly thirty thousand patients. Even then, mortality was thought to be infrequent enough that the primary endpoint for the ICU study was the combination of persistent kidney dysfunction, need for dialysis, and death. This composite outcome was also a secondary endpoint in the non-ICU study. Both studies found a statistically significant 1% absolute difference in this outcome, favoring alternative fluids compared to saline. Almost overnight, hospitals began to stock the alternative fluids in their ICUs and emergency departments alongside saline. Unfortunately, the alternative fluids could not completely replace saline because saline is still used to deliver most medication, which haven't been tested when mixed in the alternative fluids. Still, it seemed like a major victory.

---

[1] GH Evevans, "The Abuse of Normal Salt Solution," *JAMA* LVII, no. 27 (1911): 2126–2127. https://doi.org/10.1001/jama.1911.04260120316010.

But not everyone was convinced. The Vanderbilt trials were conducted at one institution and didn't randomize individual patients but instead randomized by month and by unit. While it's very unlikely this could have affected the outcome, patient-level randomization is always preferred. While the price difference between the fluids in question is fairly small, only two to three dollars per liter or about ten dollars per patient, there are over thirty-three million hospital admissions per year in the US. Thus, this change does amount to over three hundred million dollars across the entire US health-care system. While this is only about 0.02% of the $1.2 trillion annual US hospital spending, it would be a larger proportion for developing countries. Thus, a team of physician-scientists in Brazil wanted to see if the same results could be generated there. Drs. Fernando Zampieri and Alexandre Biasi Cavalvanti from the University of São Paulo led a large group of investigators throughout Brazil to enroll and randomize more than ten thousand patients to receive saline or balanced fluids. Mortality at ninety days was 26.4% for patients receiving balanced solutions and 27.2% for those receiving saline. This difference was not statistically significant but, again, was nearly 1% different. A similar trial in Australia was stopped at just over five thousand patients with the difference in mortality even smaller, about 0.2%. However, the authors of these two trials together with the Vanderbilt investigators pooled their data along with other trials and concluded that there was over a 90% chance that balanced fluids resulted in better survival compared to saline.

So do all physicians now use balanced fluids instead of saline? Amazingly, they do not. When the results of the Australian trial and a combined, so-called meta-analysis, study were published, I was asked to sit on a panel to discuss the results.[2] One of the other panelists was Dr. Jeffrey Drazen who was the editor in chief at *New England Journal of Medicine* when the Vanderbilt trials were published in that journal. Dr. Drazen noted that the trials had an immediate impact on clinical practice and noted that the shelf in his ICU that once held saline was now stocked with balanced fluids. I was happy to hear this, but then he said something else. He said that this was an important decision, but it wasn't the most important decision. Of course, he is right when it comes to an individual patient. Using the right antibiotic in a patient with an infection is likely to have a larger effect on survival. Making the right diagnosis is likely even more impactful. However, I told Dr. Draven that I disagreed with him because the decision as to what fluid to use impacts *every* patient we care for. If the difference in survival is 1%, it means that if I care for two thousand patients in a year, twenty will live or die as a result of this decision. At that point, I'd been practicing intensive care medicine for more than twenty-five years. That's five hundred patients. Even if the true effect is only half this (and it could actually be larger), it's still a large number of patients. And I'm just one doctor.

This example illustrates an important paradox. We, doctors, are motivated to do things we believe have a large effect on the patient we have in front of us even when those things are costly and time-consuming. However, we are not very good about the little things that impact all patients. This may be why, historically, doctors have been notoriously bad about washing our hands. It's only been in the last ten or twenty years that doctors have systematically complied with handwashing requirements at levels approaching acceptable even

---

[2]   https://vimeo.com/669221010.

though medical science has proven its importance as early as the late nineteenth century. Hospitals have important roles to play in filling this gap and are usually responsible for ensuring that these kinds of details are not missed. However, if hospitals have a built-in financial conflict of interest, can they really be in charge? Given the subjective nature about judging value, do we really want hospital executives to control these decisions?

CHAPTER 9

Is There a Solution?

It is difficult to get a man to understand something when his salary depends upon his not understanding it.

—Upton Sinclair

Before we examine potential solutions, let's review the problems we are seeking to solve. First, fee-for-service and "more pay for more treatment" created incentives for physicians and hospitals to do more and charge more. It's usually very easy for doctors to convince themselves and one another that a patient needs more therapy, testing, etc. After all, physicians are trained to diagnose and treat. Until relatively recently, doctors received no training on cost containment, and even today, their training is woefully inadequate. Similarly, there are no classes in medical school about the business of medicine. Furthermore, the US largely uses the tort system to resolve disputes over quality of care. Doctors can be sued in this country for virtually anything, and failure to diagnose and failure to treat are common complaints. Ordering more tests, consulting specialists, and even performing some procedures can be seen as a hedge against malpractice suits should things go badly. This so-called defensive medicine has been linked to higher costs. Even when physicians are not consciously motivated by this fear, it is easy to see how it factors in. A physician is working up some vague neurologic complaints, which the physician doesn't believe are physical. However, he considers obtaining an MRI just to be sure. The physician will likely weigh the cost of the scan against the risk of missing something. If the implication of missing something is also personal for the doctor (i.e., malpractice) and the cost is not, it's easy to see how this would likely tip the balance.

Hospitals, for their part, are in exactly the same boat as physicians under a fee-for-service model. When hospitals can charge for everything they do, doing more is good business, and hospitals too, sometimes even more so, are susceptible to the same malpractice concerns. A patient comes to an emergency department with chest pain. The pain doesn't sound cardiac (related to the heart), and the patient has none of the usual risk factors for heart disease (e.g., high blood pressure, diabetes, high cholesterol), so the likelihood that this pain is a symptom of a heart condition is low—let's say 1%. Under such conditions, it might make sense to simply reassure the patient and send them home. If, on the other hand, a hospital could be sued for more than a million dollars if the patient goes home and has a heart attack, the costs of testing, which might amount to a few hundred dollars, suddenly makes financial sense. Importantly, fixing this problem is not as easy as doing away with medical malpractice. The threat of financial consequences if care is lax not only leads to overtreatment but also encourages hospitals and physicians to do things that are needed. While most may not need this incentive, some may, and removing malpractice concerns could actually worsen care and ultimately drive costs higher as expensive treatments might be required to rescue patients from neglect.

Evidence that the system we had in place in the twentieth century led to massive increases in costs is pretty easy to come by. From 1970 to 2000, national healthcare expenditures as a percentage of GDP in the US increased 5.5%, from 7% to 12.5%. At this point, government efforts to control costs were getting serious; and over the next decade, they increased nearly another 4%, representing the largest increase relative to GDP in the nation's history. Today, they exceed 20%; but in 2019, the last "normal year" prior to the COVID-19 pandemic, they were hovering around 17%. Spending, as a percentage of GDP, had leveled off in the decade prior to the pandemic, but 17% is still a much higher number than anywhere else on the planet—nearly twice as much as the OECD member-nation average. The bargain we seem to have struck in the last decade prior to COVID-19 was that costs would be held at 17% of GDP, and hospital profits would be allowed to soar.

Unfortunately, the only way overall costs of service can be flat and profits increased is for hospital expenses to decrease, which means decreased spending on patients and their health-care providers.

If current trends continue and there is little evidence that they will change without intervention, the public can expect reduced access to innovation that does not reduce costs, a gradual deterioration in quality of healthcare, and a growing sense of dissatisfaction among providers, which will ultimately risk staffing shortages, reduced access to care, and further deterioration in care quality. This "death spiral" is all but inevitable unless we act. Conversely, a return to the "do more, charge more" model of the past would only return us to the sort of massive health-care inflation that we experienced between 1970 and 2010.

Second, we must acknowledge that corporate style healthcare did bring certain advantages just as it brought about harm. A corporate approach meant improved efficiency and integration. Access to healthcare, while still short of universal, has improved. Any reforms to our current system should not inadvertently reverse real progress. One of the biggest deficiencies of healthcare that is not based on a fee-for-service model is that there is little incentive to improve or even maintain efficiency in the system. The biggest complaints about the VA system in the US involve access to care. Although significantly improved in recent years, long waits to get into the system, to see a physician, and to schedule just about anything is, at some facilities, a nightmare. In general, when revenues are uncoupled to service, service tends to deteriorate. Healthcare is no exception. When a physician's schedule is full, "working a patient in" to such a schedule will never happen if neither the physician nor the clinic realizes any benefit. This benefit doesn't need to be financial, but if the extra work isn't even recognized, it will be very difficult to get anyone to do it.

Third, while the corporate model of healthcare has brought gains in efficiency and integration, it has not improved transparency. Hospitals are generally horrible when asked to produce an itemized bill for services provided, and when they do, they are largely fabricated. This is because hospitals are paid per diagnosis using a system of diagnosis-related groups (DRGs). So, for the hospital, it's really about documenting which DRGs their patients fall under. In fact, if the hospital really were to charge by item or service, there would at least be some accountability. However, transparency and accountability are still possible using DRGs.

Think about your last experience with servicing your car. You needed new brakes. A diagnosis-based procedure—you were noticing a sound when you applied the brakes, and an examination by a mechanic revealed the problem. The prices for new brakes are advertised and agreed on in advance of the work. Uncertainty is minimal for you and for the shop. No one does a brake job or an oil change and runs into "complications." A shop that advertises a forty-five-dollar oil change and then charges six hundred dollars because it encountered problems with your oil pressure wouldn't stay in business for long. Similarly, you don't get a bill that is higher or lower than agreed because it took longer or oil prices changed. All of this is factored into the price up front.

While it's true that medicine is far more complicated than automotive maintenance, many procedures are pretty routine—setting broken bones, appendectomies, etc. Furthermore, when you do get into a more complicated situation, the automotive shop can still provide you with an estimate. In doing so, both the payor (you) and the shop assume some risks. The transmission repair actually went much easier than expected and was finished in half the time, but you still paid full price. Or conversely, it turned out to be much harder, but you were not charged more. In the long run, these things will likely balance out, and the shop will make the expected amount of money for the expected amount of work. Similarly, an automobile repair shop that agrees to use new parts and instead uses refurbished parts to improve its bottom line is committing fraud.

Hospitals could take a similar approach if they chose to with routine surgeries and even many standard medical admissions. Such an approach could provide a much-needed measure of predictability and transparency to the system. Hospitals could lay out their costs, item by item, service by service, and arrive at a price with a certain profit built in. They would not be allowed to then substitute cheaper items or provide less-trained clinicians because these things could be specified up front. Unfortunately, hospitals will certainly resist such changes because they currently profit greatly on uncertainty and secrecy. Under a more transparent approach, hospitals could instead expect to earn a fee for providing the service rather than secretly cutting costs and pocketing the proceeds.

Finally and most importantly, physicians have historically functioned as patient advocates. For most of us, we went to medical school so we could learn how to help patients. I'm not suggesting that we don't want to be paid well to do it, far from it, but virtually, all physicians would prefer to make money in a therapeutic alliance with patients rather than being part of a system that purports to put patient care first but actually enriches hospital executives *and* physicians largely by cutting corners and trying not to harm patients in the process. Trust in the medical system is already taxed, in part as a consequence of the COVID-19 pandemic. However, overall trust in the system has been eroding for some time.

In 2014, Blendon and coworkers noted in an article in the *New England Journal of Medicine* that in 1966, 73% of Americans said they had great confidence in the leaders of the medical profession. In 2012, only 34% felt the same way. Notably, according to the same article, the US ranks twenty-fourth in the world for overall trust in

US doctors yet third in patient satisfaction with *their own* doctors. A 2021 study conducted at the request of the American Board of Internal Medicine found that nearly one in three physicians surveyed (30%) say their trust in the US health-care system and health-care organization leadership has decreased over the prior year. Only 18% report increased trust. This is in stark contrast to the overwhelming trust physicians have in their fellow clinicians. Physicians report high levels of trust for other physicians and nurses (88%) while only two-thirds (66%) trust health-care organization leaders and executives. These attitudes closely match those of patients. Trust in doctors (84%) and nurses (85%) is high while trust in the health-care system as a whole is far lower (64%). About one in three patients (32%) say their trust in the health-care system decreased during the pandemic, compared to 11% whose trust increased.

Of perhaps even greater significance, mistrust of physicians seems to be largely driven by factors like a lack of time spent with patients and not directly related to concerns for financial conflict of interest. Only 8% of patients said they mistrusted their doctors because they were too financially motivated. This fact seems telling. Few health-care consumers, it seems, appreciate how much financial motivations might be influencing physician decisions. Interestingly, only 10% of physicians felt that mistrust in them was a function of economic self-interest. This may well indicate that physicians are themselves only dimly aware of the influence the system has on their behavior.

Another interesting statistic is that patients have low trust in health insurance companies (33%) and physicians even lower (19%). This is interesting in part because some insurance companies own and operate hospitals and clinics. This arrangement is called an integrated health delivery system, and Kaiser Permanente is the best known. In fact, Kaiser is the largest not-for-profit health maintenance organization in the US. Headquartered in Oakland, California, the organization serves 8.2 million members in nine states and the District of Columbia. The Kaiser system includes the health plans, the hospitals, and the Permanente Medical Groups (doctors and offices). The three groups cooperate under mutually exclusive contracts to provide one-stop health-care services. Interestingly, Kaiser is possibly the most well-liked system by patients, routinely achieving high patient satisfaction for all three arms of the organization.

The concern with an integrated health delivery system is that all utilization can be controlled centrally. In essence, Kaiser and organizations like it have full control over what drugs they use, what staffing ratios are maintained in the hospital, and what they pay their staff. In turn, patients are at the mercy of the system with just the sort of potential conflicts of interest that we have been discussing, except that it's all one organization. Is this good or bad? It appears to be difficult to say. On the one hand, a health maintenance organization that works with a number of different hospitals can seek the best value across multiple options, whereas in a single integrated system, there is no choice. On the other hand, if an HMO contract is designed to generate revenue for the HMO and hospitals engage in such contracts with their own revenue calculations, you have, in reality, two organizations (the insurer and the provider) looking to make money. With an integrated system, you can cut the number of organizations in half. The company's "not-for-profit" status is certainly no guarantee that it won't be profiting.

In 2021, even in the throes of the COVID-19 pandemic, Kaiser Foundation Health Plan (KFHP) posted "earnings" of only $307,000 dollars, but Kaiser also paid forty-five million dollars to its top executives or, more aptly, they kept forty-five million dollars for themselves. Not bad especially when you consider that they also reported an average of only 21.2 hours of work per week for each of the ten executives.

It is often stated, usually by executives, that executive salary is not really an issue in terms of the overall economics of an organization. Indeed, Kaiser employs more than twenty-three thousand doctors and more than sixty-five thousand nurses. Even if they were to use the forty-five million dollars to increase clinician salaries, it would only result in a two-thousand dollar raise per doctor or seven hundred dollars per nurse. Alternatively, this amount could be used to hire an additional 150–200 doctors or roughly five hundred nurses, neither of which is greater than 1% of the workforce. However, these numbers are better used to illustrate that in a system this large, you only need to cut about 1% of the workforce to save forty-five million dollars. It's how these organizations can squeeze large sums out of the workforce with relatively small-appearing changes. Similarly, cutting a benefit worth only a few hundred dollars per nurse is able to generate twenty million dollars across the system. Given these economics, it's easy to see how health-care executives have become addicted to workforce austerity as a means of generating large sums to pay for lost revenues elsewhere in the system and, yes, to pay for outrageous executive compensation as well.

Examining Kaiser's executive pay from a different perspective, the forty-five million dollars we just discussed only costs each insured patient about five dollars a year, so doing away with executive compensation or cutting it back to something reasonable isn't going to save much money for patients. The problem instead is that once established, these costs become fixed in the system and become expectations. If, in the future, Kaiser was projecting a forty-five-million-dollar shortfall, doing away with executive salaries for the year wouldn't be on the table. Instead, the management team would weigh increasing premiums or cutting costs. Increasing premiums, even slightly within a contract year, is usually impossible, so taking the forty-five million dollars out of the doctor or nurse salary pool, for example, by just delaying new hires that were set to fill open positions by a few months would actually do the trick. Alternatively, pulling forty-five million dollars out of a five- or six-billion-dollar pharmacy budget is usually doable in any given year. Whichever approach is taken, patients will be disadvantaged, if only slightly, and executive compensation will be protected. This is the essence of the underlying conflict of interest we've been examining in this book.

Given all the risk and very real conflicts of interest inherent in a system that employs physicians, one might ask, Is it really a good idea? Until very recently, physician practices were mostly independent of hospitals. Even in hospital-based specialties, like anesthesia and emergency medicine, doctors were not uniformly employees of the hospital system that they worked in but instead were either independent or, more commonly, belonged to a private group practice. As discussed in chapter 6, this arrangement has multiple downsides for physicians, the most important being financial security. Over the last three to four decades, physicians have been choosing, more and more, to take the financial security of a hospital employer over the autonomy of an independent practice or practice group because of the uncertainty inherent in owning their own practices. Unfortunately, for patients, they no longer have an independent advocate in their doctor. But did they ever really have one? In the fee-for-service environment of the late twentieth century and extending in some ways to the present, a doctor's financial self-interest could still be entangled in their clinical decision-making. A surgeon who does an operation or a cardiologist who performs a heart procedure will make more money compared to when they advise the patient *not* to have these treatments.

So is the physician as objective advocate just an illusion? One way to examine this question is to consider how these potential conflicts of interest are managed and how transparent they are. The laws against self-referral that were discussed in chapter 5, the very ones that the government is currently dismantling in the name of value-based care, were designed to deal with this very issue. If a doctor recommends that you have your gallbladder removed and he or she also earns more money if you have the operation than if you don't, then there is an incentive to recommend the surgery. If, on the other hand, the doctor has no financial stake in the process because the surgeon performing the operation and the hospital in which it is performed are not connected to the referring doctor, then the doctor has no financial stake in the treatment. Second opinions, prevalent from the 1950s to the 1980s, also served to provide an objective assessment. The doctor providing the second opinion could not benefit in any way from the outcome and, therefore, could be more objective. Of course, neither system is perfect, but the point is that systems have developed over many years to at least address the concern.

No such system, apart from whistleblower protection, is in place to reduce the impact of employer-based conflict of interest. Indeed, just the opposite. CMS and other payors seem to be quite happy to have some conflicts as long as costs are controlled.

A second point is that direct financial conflicts of interest for doctors are very transparent and tend to be scrutinized. A cardiologist who performs heart procedures like angioplasty on patients that his or her peers do not tends to stick out. This is not to say that some physicians do not flaunt the norms of their profession, and many get away with it for years. For example, a cancer surgeon who operates on patients with disease so advanced that most other surgeons would not will likely do more cases. Doing more cases brings in more revenue for the hospital and, therefore, gives the surgeon some measure of power within the organization. This power can be used to effectively silence any objections to the surgeon's aggressive practice. Eventually, these sorts of arrangements fall apart, but they can persist for many years and are frequently out in the open. However, these kinds of practices are usually the exceptions. Medical schools teach ethics using these kinds of examples, and patients are not usually mystified by the financial relationships between recommending a procedure and getting paid to do it. By contrast, patients are generally unaware about the extent to which employer-based conflicts of interest can influence clinician practices toward doing less or spending less, and these decisions have serious potential to impact their care.

Thus, one policy change that would seem critical is to make it impossible for hospitals and insurance companies to employ doctors. If doctors were all independent and could work directly for patients, a major source of conflict of interest would be eliminated. Other safeguards would also be necessary to prevent coercion by the system (such as the recently enacted legislation addressing surprise billing), but doctors could return to their traditional roles as advocates for their patients. An alternative system would be to have independent patient advocates available for patients, but since these people would most likely have to be doctors themselves, such a system would be very expensive even if we had enough physicians in the country, which we don't. We also have to accept that disentangling physician practices from hospitals would almost certainly increase costs. The practice consolidations seen over the last thirty years were motivated by a desire to reduce costs. Independent physicians tend to prescribe therapies that are best for their patients rather than for the hospital bottom line. However, hospital profits are large and can certainly absorb some increased costs. They are also quite expert in cost containment, and when dealing with patients, the relationship is completely lopsided in terms of power. Putting physicians back in the patients' corner is essential to deal with this power dynamic.

Importantly, a handful of states already have statutes that prohibit the direct employment of doctors by hospitals. For example, the California Medical Practice Act or, more specifically, the Business and Professions Code (B&P) Section 2052 states that practicing medicine without a valid license is unlawful. Medical licenses are issued only to individuals, not to businesses. Advocates cite the need to prevent corporate interference with the practice of medicine as the primary reason for this prohibition. If corporations can dictate how patients are treated, it opens the door to conflicts between patients' interests and the hospitals' business interests.

One of the primary opponents to hospitals employing doctors is the California Medical Association. On their website under the Top Issue, "Physician-Patient Relationship," they state the following:

> The California Medical Association (CMA) fiercely defends California's bar on the corporate practice of medicine, which prevents corporate interests from unduly influencing physicians' professional judgments in the name of profit and to the detriment of patients.
>
> Hospitals and other corporate interests do not have the same ethical and moral obligation to the patient as a physician does; therefore, it is essential to maintain the firewall between medical decisions and the corporate bottom line.
>
> CMA also leads efforts in multiple arenas to leave the determination of what is medically necessary treatment where it belongs—in the hands of doctors. Health insurance gatekeepers and finance officers continually find new ways to delay and deny care, and erect barriers to medically necessary care for patients.

This "firewall" between hospitals' interests and patients' interests and between health insurer interests and patients' interest is precisely what we are talking about. Ironically, while California prohibits a hospital or a corporation from directly hiring physicians, it neither prevents the existence of large physician practice groups nor the formation of an integrated delivery system (IDS). Indeed, Kaiser Permanente, one the first and possibly the best-known examples of an IDS, is headquartered in Oakland, California, and the majority of its business is in California.

Across the US, there are a growing number of IDSs and other forms of affiliation between doctors, hospitals, and insurance companies. With the advent of Accountable Care Organizations under the Affordable Care Act, we will see even more collaboration between these three sectors of our healthcare system in the future. Without major corrective action and current trends in so-called health-care reform are in the opposite direction, the doctor-hospital firewall that still exists in a few states will crumble. Not only is corrective action needed but it's also needed now. As Ezekiel Emanuel, MD puts it in his book *Which Country Has the World's Best Healthcare:*[3] "healthcare is path-dependent," meaning that we cannot ignore the effects of preexisting institutional structures on the trajectory of reform. The longer the current trends continue, the more intrenched they will become. If we want to change the course of health-care evolution in this country, we need to act now.

Other approaches might also be considered. Socialized medicine or a one-payor system could also remove the profit motive, but as we see from experience with those systems in other countries or our own VA system, new problems may be encountered. In the end, physician independence from the system they work in is essential to limiting employer-based conflict of interest and serves to align physicians with the patients they care for. More regulations may also

---

[3] Ezekiel "Zeke" Emanuel, MD, *Which Country Has the World's Best Healthcare?* (Public Affairs Press, 2020).

have a role, but so far, government has been mainly concerned with reducing costs. Some reforms may actually cost more, but society should be able to have input into whether it perceives value rather than being told what a value-based system is.

CHAPTER 10

What Can We, as Health-Care Consumers, Do until a Solution Is Found?

Unless someone like you cares a whole awful lot,
nothing is going to get better. It's not.

—Dr. Seuss

Given the magnitude of the problems inherent in US health-care, it would be understandable, as a patient, to feel overwhelmed and helpless. Many of the problems discussed in this book are structural. How can any one of us change the structure of US healthcare? Actually, there is a lot we can do. My recipe for patient activism is similar to the strategies I use when dealing with my own health-care system. Of course, I'm a physician and have held senior positions within the health-care system I use for many years. You would expect that it would be easier for me. In truth, I think it is a lot easier, but this neither means that I don't encounter some of the same problems as everyone nor does it mean that the strategies I use can't be used by others. My strategy has four parts:

1. Exercising choice where we can (e.g., doctor, health insurer).
2. Seek alternatives and comparison shop. Prenegotiate whenever you can.
3. Ask to see the details. Don't just accept what you are told, and don't just accept what you are charged.
4. Take political action (emphasis on fairness and transparency, not financing models per se).

Exercising Choice

Another unfortunate consequence of the physician shortage in the US, discussed in chapter 3, is that in many communities, it's hard to find a doctor. In most urban centers, there is a mix of independent practices and corporate practices, the latter rapidly overtaking the former. Independent, physician-owned practices routinely stop taking new patients when they reach some level, determined largely by physician preferences. They may then start taking new patients again if the numbers in the practice fall. Corporate practices, by contrast, will often continue to take patients, usually resulting in long wait times for new appointments, crowded schedules, shorter visits, more use of physician extenders, etc. The physician shortage creates high demand and, thus, allows corporate practices to get away with these "inconveniences." Many patients simply don't have a choice. The system is also self-perpetuating. A corporate practice that overschedules will bring in more money at the expense of patient satisfaction and even, in some cases, outcomes. However, if new patients are desperate, the low satisfaction won't be much of factor. Then the practice can entice new doctors at a higher salary or buy up independent practices and continue to overschedule.

A system that buys a practice from two retiring doctors might only hire one new doctor to replace them. They can pay the new doctor a bit more and still make a larger profit—never mind that the patients in the practice will now experience a dramatic change in their care experience. It's very likely that this helps to explain why the US gets low marks for overall trust in doctors (twenty-fourth in the world) while it ranks third in patient satisfaction with individuals' own doctors. Patients generally like and trust doctors they have but are suspicious and unhappy with a system that is gradually becoming more impersonal and much less user-friendly.

We can see similar trends playing out in Europe. A study from 2014 on patient satisfaction in seven European countries found that Germany had the lowest satisfaction at 59.5%, and Italy had the highest at 87.4%. One factor in this could be that Germany has half as many doctors per population as Italy. You might be shocked to learn that the ability to choose your physician is actually lower in the US than in many other countries. Insurance companies in the US are exercising more and more control over which doctors we can see. So-called health-care reform isn't helping. Managed competition, a strategy for health-care delivery whereby costs are reduced by fostering competition between providers of managed-care contracts, is a popular strategy among health-care policy experts. For managed competition to work, closed networks of hospital and providers are needed, and this limits choice. Americans are used to experiencing situations where a physician of their choice no longer accepts their insurance. However, modern managed competition can take this to a higher level where the physician can't accept the patient's insurance even if they wanted to. Physician fees for office visits are a small fraction of the costs the insurance company is seeking to control. Indeed, your preferred doctor might even cost less. However, the insurer also wants the physician to prescribe less-expensive therapy. In ideal situations, this is scientific and rational. Two drugs have the same benefit and same side-effect profile, but the insurer has negotiated a better price for one of them. However, just as often, the situation is not ideal. The drugs don't have exactly the same benefits or the same risks, and it's a judgment call as to whether the cost difference is worth it.

As we've seen time and again, when these decisions are left to doctors' advice and patients' pocketbooks, a range of choices are made, just as we can observe with orders for food at our favorite restaurant. I like lobster and will occasionally splurge for it while my wife thinks it tastes like chicken and will not. Naproxen (brand name Aleve) and ibuprofen (one common brand name is Motrin) are very similar nonsteroidal anti-inflammatory drugs that have virtually identical effectiveness and safety profiles. If you take one of these drugs regularly for, say, arthritis pain, a one-month supply of naproxen will cost about $11.67 or thirty-nine cents per day. Motrin costs slightly more at about $16.97 for a one-month supply or about fifty-seven cents per day. To most but not all patients, the price difference is trivial, and factors like ease of use, number of doses required each day, or even the taste of the pill will be the only factors we consider. For some patients, ibuprofen is preferred because you can take it more often whereas other patients will prefer naproxen precisely because you don't need to take it as often. However, if you are a large insurance provider with a million patients taking one or the other of these drugs, $5.30 per month price difference amounts to $63.6 million per year. For this money, the insurer will almost certainly consider issues like convenience or the taste of pills inconsequential.

Even larger cost differences may exist between prescription medications, and these are the ones that your insurance company may be trying to control. Of course, the insurer can simply restrict drugs on its plan or charge a higher co-payment for drugs it pays more for, but patients notice and, indeed, may become very frustrated when they find out that a drug that their doctor has prescribed isn't covered by their insurance plan. By contrast, if the insurer can control the prescribing in the first place, patients may not even know that there are alternatives.

Even if your insurer isn't restricting your choice of doctor, you may be restricted by the supply of doctors in your community. There is considerable variation in the supply of physicians across the US. According to a 2017 AAMC State Physician Workforce Data Report, there are three states with fewer than two physicians per one thousand population: Mississippi, Idaho, and Wyoming. Nevada isn't much better with exactly two per one thousand. Furthermore, there are twenty-two states, including some very populous ones, such as Texas that have fewer than 2.5 physicians per one thousand population. Meanwhile, Massachusetts boasts 4.4, and four others, Rhode Island, Vermont, Maryland, and New York, all have more than 3.5. Thus, the probability of finding a doctor who is taking new patients is roughly twice as high if you live in Maryland compared to Mississippi. Of course, other factors are also important. Rural communities tend to have fewer physicians per capita, and poor and minority communities are most disadvantaged.

If you are fortunate enough to live in a community that has several physician practices to choose from, you will likely want to consider several factors before deciding which one to use. Even if you don't have many choices, it's a good idea to consider these factors and discuss them with the physician that you see. The odds are good that the doctor you encounter will not have been asked these questions very often and may well react with surprise and possibly annoyance. Still, it's a good idea to have these conversations before deciding to use their services. First, who owns the practice? If the practice is owned by a hospital system, an employer-based conflict of interest is inherent. How is this conflict of interest managed? Does the physician feel pressure to use cheaper treatments to reduce costs? What happens when the physician believes that a more expensive treatment is best for the patient? Is the physician paid bonuses for reducing costs? This last question will raise an eyebrow for sure. Few physicians will be willing to share information about their own compensation with patients, but how they react to this question may indeed be telling. A physician who reacts with compassion and reassurance could be lying, but most will simply refuse to answer or become angry if they are, in fact, receiving payments from their employers specifically based on saving money.

If you want to take a less direct approach, you may want to ask about how disputes are settled and whether physicians are involved in the governance of the practice even if they don't own it. However, as we've discussed, physician input into the decision-making is not a guarantee that decisions will be made on the basis of what's best for patients. This is the whole nature of the conflict of interest. Is the physician really able to put your interests ahead of all others?

Just as importantly, if the doctors own their own practice, what else do they own? Do the physicians have a stake in a medical imaging, pathology, or laboratory services company? As discussed in chapter 5, referral to these centers by doctors with an ownership stake is against the law. However, there are communities where this still happens in open defiance of the law. Furthermore, these laws are being scaled back in the name of value-based healthcare.

Understanding how the doctors are compensated may not seem like any of your business as a patient, but you are entitled to know if financial relationships are in place that could compromise your care. The employer-sponsored health insurance system, which still insures more than half of all Americans, actually obscures accountability. Most Americans think of this as a benefit; indeed, health coverage is called a benefit by employers and tax accountants alike. However, workers pay for this insurance in three ways. First, a portion of the insurance premiums are paid by the employees directly, and there are usually some co-payments or deductibles. Second, economists have demonstrated that, on average, employer-sponsored health insurance reduces wages, so, in effect, the employer doesn't pay; we do. Finally, in 1954, Congress enacted a tax exclusion on health-care benefits from payroll taxes. This tax exemption amounts to more than three hundred billion dollars a year and is the single largest tax exemption in the United States. This is three hundred billion dollars that the treasury has to make up with other taxes, so, again, we are paying for it. The next time you see "benefits" on your pay stub, think about this.

The next question to ask a physician you are considering is what happens when you are hospitalized? Will your physician, who understands your values and preferences, see you in the hospital? Chances are she won't. Whereas twenty years ago this was the norm, today, few physicians practicing in outpatient settings see patients in the hospital. Will someone from the same practice see you? Some physician groups have "hospitalists," physicians caring for patients in the hospital, and work alongside their ambulatory partners to coordinate care. However, this is not the majority. In many communities, care is fragmented and chaotic between outpatient and inpatient care. In the worst cases, hospitalists don't even have access to outpatient records; and when patients are discharged back to their outpatient providers, the physicians can't directly access the hospital records instead rely on summaries that are sent to them by mail!

More and more information is available online for products or services we might wish to use. Unfortunately, the accuracy of these data can be quite limited. The website health.usnews.com correctly identifies the hospital I work at but has me listed as a pulmonologist (lung disease specialist). It doesn't show any patient reviews. The site doctor.webmd.com, by contrast, correctly lists me as a critical care specialist but not the right hospital. It lists ratings from only two patients. Still, it's worth looking to see if a prospective physician or office practice has lots of positive or negative reviews or whether they have been in the news for the right or the wrong reasons.

A recent development in physician practice is so-called "concierge medicine." This is a private practice arrangement where patients can pay an annual fee to have much greater access to a physician's services. Like a retainer for a law firm, the contract gives the patient preferred access to the practice. For example, some concierge medicine providers give patients their cell phone numbers and make house calls. They will see patients on weekends, and because they typically have dramatically fewer patients, there is usually a way to work the patient in if there is an urgent need. At its inception, concierge medicine was expensive and really only for the wealthy. Fees were typically $150–$200 per month ($1,800–$2,400 per year), some significantly more and could offer some pretty "white-glove" style services. However, less-expensive models for primary care have emerged and are taking root in many communities.

According to market analyses, the concierge medicine market is growing rapidly and is expected to double over the next six to eight years. Concierge medicine still gets mixed reviews from some patients and from industry analysts. However, most patients, including the ones whom I've spoken to, seem quite pleased. The website medicalecomonics.com runs regular articles on the topic. Models seem to vary greatly, with some charging a very modest annual fee but only providing a small change in service. Others, at higher fees, dramatically change the experience.

Consider the economics. A busy general internist might have a practice with 2,500 or even 3,000 patients. If the chronic disease burden in the practice is even modestly high, the average patient might see their doctor four or five times or more a year. Let's say the average is only three. That's upward of nine thousand visits a year. In the US, the average year has about 260 working days, and if you back out four weeks of vacation, a physician might be seeing patients 220 days a year. That's forty patients a day or one every ten minutes over an eight-hour day. If ten minutes sounds quite rushed and, surely, it is, try doing the math differently.

There are only a few ways to accomplish this, and the most common is to use physician extenders (e.g., nurse practitioners) to see most of the annual checkups and even some of the sick visits. If a primary care doctor is seeing this many patients, they may be making more than average, perhaps three hundred thousand dollars per year in salary and another seventy-five thousand dollars in benefits. This effectively means that they are paid about forty-two dollars a visit or about $125 a year for every patient in their practice. If that doesn't sound like very much, then you get the appeal of concierge medicine.

If the physician were to reduce their practice to only one thousand patients and charge them all $250 per year retainer or roughly a quarter of the average annual health club membership, he could see far fewer patients in a day (two-thirds fewer) and potentially spend thirty minutes with each of them. He would need to cover overhead too, but he would no longer need a physician extender. So let's say he charges $375 per year (still less than half of a health club membership) and makes his annual salary just from the retainer, using the revenue from the three thousand office visits per year to pay for his now reduced overhead. He could even provide discounts for annual checkups, and the physician would still make more money, work less, and have happier and, possibly, healthier patients.

Given these economics, it's easy to see how concierge medicine would be popular with patients and providers alike. Some physicians express feelings of guilt, though, about limiting their practices when there are already so few doctors. However, most experience such an increase in patient satisfaction that concerns are rapidly alleviated. The fact that many families might find it difficult to pay such fees for four or five members is a concern, but $375 per person out of the annual family health-care budget is relatively small for most. Some people choose health-care insurance plans that have only a thirty- or forty-dollar co-payment for office visits and may pay thousands of dollars a year for the coverage. Most would be better off with a less-expensive plan that didn't cover office visits at all, putting the money instead in a concierge medicine fee with higher charges per visit. It might actually be more economical for many.

However, if you are considering concierge medicine, make sure you have a complete understanding of what you are getting and how much it will cost. Some concierge medicine practices still charge very high rates, and some have affordable rates but offer little real benefit. I haven't actually found one that charges as low as the $375 per year that I've used as an illustration above. One reason is that growth in concierge medicine has largely been in national companies that organize the service. No doubt they are taking a large "administrative fee." The concierge medicine industry is highly unregulated, and there is certainly the potential for profiteering. If fees are more than one thousand dollars per year, practice sizes should be very small, say less than four hundred to five hundred, or else the fees should include some of the costs that would otherwise be out of pocket.

The concierge medicine market for inpatient physician services is practically nonexistent. Some gold-plated plans, in addition to providing house calls, will include seeing you in the hospital, but this is not typical. However, given the growth in the concierge medicine market, it's likely that services will continue to expand, and care models will continue to evolve.

A second area where we can sometimes exercise choice is with our insurance plan. Most Americans don't shop very much or very well for health insurance. Roughly a third of Medicare recipients have selected Medicare Advantage, which provides them with additional benefits but may also leave them with expensive co-payments. Many would actually be better off having stayed with traditional Medicare. For employer-sponsored health insurance, there is a tendency to value coverage for lower-cost services we will use more than higher-cost services we may or may not use.

For example, people will pay higher premiums if physician visits are "covered" because they know they will see a physician at least once a year. However, this really isn't insurance. It's more akin to a payday loan. If you are paying a monthly insurance premium to reduce your out-of-pocket charges for the inevitable visit to the doctor, then you are just shifting costs and possibly not in your favor. Many plans charge over one thousand dollars per year to cover physician office visits, and there are still co-payments. A primary care office visit might cost two hundred dollars and a specialist three hundred dollars. With insurance, you may still be charged co-payments of thirty to forty dollars. So unless you expect to see a specialist twice and a primary care provider three times in a single year, you'd actually be better off without this insurance.

Conversely, many people opt out of plans that cover less common but very expensive care. Does your plan cover air ambulance services? These services can cost tens of thousands, and insurance coverage is usually available within the insurance plans offered by most major carriers. Most Americans don't have long-term care coverage, yet many of us will need long-term care at some point, and it's very expensive. This sort of protection is what insurance is for. Office visit coverage and most prescription drug benefits are not insurance. They are cost-shifting schemes, and most are not cost-effective.

Most insurance plans now offer coverage for prescription drugs. Almost everyone purchasing these plans uses prescription drugs, so it's not an insurance that distributes risk. Sure, some recipients will need more or higher-cost drugs compared to others, but what is really going on here? As discussed in chapter 2, the insurance market for pharmacy benefits is complex and convoluted. Most insurance companies hire pharmacy benefit managers (PBMs), essentially middlemen in the prescription drug marketplace, to manage the pharmacy benefits for their patients. PBMs buy drugs wholesale and then charge the insurer, often at an exorbitant markup. Because fees, discounts, and rebates affect the prices PBMs pay for drugs, it's usually impossible to know the difference between what they are being charged and what the PBMs actually paid for each drug. As a result, health insurance companies are now collaborating with PBMs and even own them in many cases, such as United Health and Optima X, Cigna and Express Scripts, and Aetna and CVS Care Mart. You may be paying for a prescription drug benefit, but in some cases, you may not be the one benefiting. Through their PBMs, insurers are negotiating deep discounts on certain drugs and then claiming the discount as an insurance benefit. For example, a PBM may be able to purchase a common drug like simvastatin (a cholesterol lowering drug) for twenty cents per twenty-milligram tablet. They can then fill a prescription for you for ninety tablets and only charge you a thirty-dollar co-payment.

This will seem like a good deal because your local CVS will quote you a $56.69 cost for this prescription. However, the PBM is only paying eighteen dollars for the drug. So in effect, the insurance company is charging you a monthly premium for the ability to overcharge you.

Now if the PBM cannot negotiate as good a price for alternative drugs in the same class, for example, atorvastatin and fluvastatin, they may tell you that these drugs are not covered under your plan. You might then go online and find that you can get ninety tablets of atorvastatin for only twenty-five dollars through GoodRx, for example. You might even cancel your prescription drug coverage altogether. However, if the insurance company can also dictate which doctors you can see, they can ensure that you'll be getting prescriptions for the drugs they want you to use and possibly locking you into paying for them twice: once for the premium and then again for each prescription. And you may well think that you got a good deal in the process. Doctors, for their parts, may have little insight into this scheme. To them, your insurance doesn't allow atorvastatin and fluvastatin, and there is really no medical evidence that they are superior to simvastatin. Unless you were to ask them (and why would you?), it's unlikely that the choice of drug would even be discussed.

Seek Alternatives and Comparison Shop

Any interaction with the health-care marketplace should be approached with caution and an eye toward finding the best deal. Prices and outcomes for routine surgeries, such as hip replacements and cataract surgery, can vary widely even in the same city. Let's say you have Medicare, and there are six hospitals in your area that can perform these procedures. The cost to you will be the same, so the choice should be based on quality. Do your research, starting with your primary care doctor, but also speak with friends and relatives who had the same procedures. Look online but be careful to check the sources. If you have Medicare Advantage, you may be responsible for a co-payment. Check with your insurance carrier first. Some co-payments are calculated on the total bill where you pay a percentage. Others are based on standard pricing. If the hospital charges more, you may be responsible for all or part of the excess. In both cases, a less-expensive hospital may end up costing you less.

For prescription drugs, Consumer Reports recommends three steps. First, use online discounts—GoodRx, Link Health, WeRx.org all show pricing at various locations and offer online discounts. If pushed, most pharmacies will honor them. Ask before you hand the prescription over. At a grocery store chain pharmacy in California, I asked and was told no, but when I turned to leave, I was stopped and asked to wait until a supervisor could be consulted. Ultimately, they accepted the coupon. In some cases, it may be better to not use your insurance. Ask for all available discounts and see if using insurance is really the best deal. You'll get odd looks from the cashier, but then when the insurance price is actually higher, you will be vindicated. Also, don't just use the big-box stores. HealthWarehouse.com, Costco, and Sam's Club may seem like the best value, as they are for many things, but try to use independent pharmacies whenever possible. You'll often get better pricing and better service.

Finally, you may be surprised to learn that you can prenegotiate most nonemergent care. Few people actually do this, but you really can. That knee replacement might cost you as much as a vacation in Europe, and that's with insurance. You'd be crazy not to try and get a better price. If you contact your insurance provider, you might learn that having the procedure at one hospital will be 100% covered, while at another, it's not.

Ask to See the Details

Unfortunately, the above steps will not always be possible. Emergencies do happen, and you may well find yourself having to accept what is being offered. However, you should not just accept what you are told and definitely not accept what you are charged without a complete explanation. In his book[4] *The Price We Pay*, Marty Makary, MD describes an experience with a friend who required emergency medical care while she was visiting from out of town. She was "out of network" and warned that her insurance may not pay for the visit. As expected, his friend was given the usual forms to sign in which a patient consents to treatment *and* agrees to pay 100% of whatever the hospital decides to charge. Most patients sign these forms. Indeed, they are usually put together into one form so they appear to be interdependent. With one signature, the patient agrees to both treatment and an open-ended contract to pay.

The problem is that obtaining emergency care and agreeing to pay are actually separated by law. In 1986, Congress enacted the Emergency Medical Treatment and Labor Act (EMTALA) to ensure public access to emergency services regardless of ability to pay. Section 1867 of the Social Security Act imposes specific obligations

---

[4]　Marty Makary, MD, *The Price We Pay: What Broke American Health Care—and How to Fix It* (Bloomsbury Publishing, 2019).

on Medicare-participating hospitals that offer emergency services to provide a medical screening examination when a request is made for one or treatment for an emergency medical condition, including active labor, regardless of an individual's ability to pay. Hospitals are then required to provide stabilizing treatment for patients with emergency medical conditions. If a hospital is unable to stabilize a patient within its capability or if the patient requests, an appropriate transfer should be implemented.

Makary goes on to say that when his friend was given this form, it was on an iPad so it could not even be modified. He requested a paper form for her so the language concerning a blank check to the hospital could be crossed out. His friend consented to be treated but did not agree to pay whatever the hospital asked. She was then evaluated, admitted, and received a routine surgical procedure. She recovered fully and went home. The inflated charges for the out-of-network care were staggering. Fortunately, his foresight to refuse an open-ended payment allowed for the bill to be negotiated.

Even if a contract is in place, there may still be room to negotiate. However, it won't be pretty. The usual place to start is with an itemized bill. This sounds straightforward, but it rarely is. Hospitals must provide such bills if requested, but they don't need to make it easy. There may be request forms and other documentation, and when the bill finally arrives, it may be hard to interpret. Parts that are usually easier to understand include pharmacy costs and surgeons' fees. These are good places to look for potential overcharges. Did you actually receive the medication you were billed for? Often, you may not know for sure, but some you may recognize. Were you billed for blood transfusions you were not told about and perhaps didn't actually receive? The surgeon who operated on you has an office. Are you seeing her in follow-up? You might want to consider discussing the bill with her. Chances are she'll have no idea what the hospital is charging you for her services. She may be willing to reduce the bill.

Under the Affordable Care Act, hospitals are required to offer financial assistance and set parameters for what hospitals can do. Even if the bill cannot be negotiated, the payment parameters usually can be. Be careful, however, as hospitals are notorious for inflating prices, only to later offer a small discount. In the case described by Marty Makary, his friend was originally charged five times the going rate and, in the end, was offered a 10% discount.

Take Political Action

A friend of mine, Claudio, a nephrologist from Italy, is an avid traveler, and he loves to shop in exotic markets in faraway lands. I was once with him in the Grand Bazaar in Istanbul, and he was looking to buy some antique pots. I went off to buy some jewelry for my wife and daughter, and when I returned, he was still haggling with the shop owner. They finally agreed on a price, and he made the purchase. As we left the store, he asked me what I purchased, and I told him along with the price I had paid.

"You paid too much!" he exclaimed.

"How do you know? You haven't even seen the pieces," I responded.

"You Americans always overpay. You need to haggle more. You are increasing the final prices for all of us."

In case you are wondering what this has to do with taking political action, the answer is nothing. But it is a way of affecting change. If most of us accept the asking price, the price will continue to go up. If we all start haggling, it will go down. If everyone just asks the price, the pricing will be more transparent.

Much of the political debate on health-care financing concerns overarching systems, like whether a single-payor system like Medicare for all would be better than the fragmented system we now have. Much of this debate concerns access rather than costs. However, the US is actually closer to universal healthcare than ever before, with nearly 92% of the population covered. Fairness and transparency in healthcare are now just as problematic as access, and these problems are actually getting worse. Recent "innovations," like Medicare Advantage, create less transparency because many don't understand that their care may now result in large out-of-pocket expenses in exchange for certain services they may not actually need.

Just as problematic, reformers all seem convinced that traditional fee-for-service has led to exorbitant health-care costs in the US and that this is mainly due to overtreatment. As such, the solution is to treat less. However, this is overly simplistic in the extreme. Healthcare in the US is twice as expensive as in other OECD countries, yet evidence for overutilization in the US is limited to perhaps 10% or 15% tops, and even this can be debated. Compared to countries with much lower costs, we don't appear to utilize more healthcare. Fee-for-service models for physician services coexist alongside publicly funded hospital systems in many OECD countries. In still others, both physicians and hospitals are private, and healthcare costs are controlled by regulating payments, not by regulating the practice of medicine. Soon, the US will have the world's first health-care corporatocracy—a system of government dominated by corporations and their business interests. We are on this path without much forethought and with little consideration for the inherent risks even though many are quite obvious. Again, we, as citizens and health-care consumers, have a voice in this discussion, but the public has largely been silent. This is to be expected, perhaps because the public is almost completely unaware of the evolving structures. Value-based healthcare sounds wonderful, but when it's rightly called "value for the health-care system," the public may begin to question the alignment with their values. This is not to suggest that the traditional fee-for-service model had patient values at its core, but we should not assume that bringing value to the health-care system will automatically benefit patients. Similarly, we might all feel we can get behind pay for performance, but if we called it "more money for doing less," would we be as enthusiastic?

As discussed in chapter 5, the underlying premise of "value-based payment arrangements" is to link payment to patient-centered outcomes. For example, providers can be paid incentives to achieve certain outcomes. This sounds like the answer to the faulty business model discussed in chapter 2. If a hospital can make more money by achieving outcomes that patients desire, everyone should win. However, what's missing from this description is that value-based care models that have been put forth are motivated first and foremost by saving money. While politicians might believe that reducing government spending on healthcare benefits us all, they are wrong if our individual costs all go up as a result. There is no magic formula where hospitals make more money and quality improves while costs to the public and private sectors go down. At best, there are trade-offs, and we, as health-care consumers, should have a voice in discussing the merits of these trade-offs.

One targeted area where public input seems critically absent concerns the decisions to roll back regulations prohibiting self-referral, so-called Stark laws. The argument is that these laws were put in place to protect the government from being overcharged, and now that the government is switching to another means of cost control, value-based payment arrangements, it no longer needs this protection. The collection of regulations that are commonly referred to as Stark laws began in 1989 as the Ethics in Patient Referrals bill. It is unclear how patient referrals will be more ethical without these regulations or what approach will be used to address the inevitable conflicts of interest that arise for integrated delivery systems.

State and local governments may have a larger role to play in managing health-care evolution than Congress. As discussed in chapter 7, there are significant differences in health-care spending and quality across state lines. It will require voters to make these issues political issues. If voters ask, "Why can't we have healthcare like…" politicians may be motivated to find answers. There may be many reasons why life expectancies are lower in one state compared to neighboring states. However, healthcare (quality, access, and affordability) is certainly an important place to look. The three states in the US with longest life expectancies are Hawaii, California, and New York, each longer than eighty-one years. The three lowest are Mississippi, West Virginia, and Alabama, all below seventy-six years. Yes, median household income might well be a large determinant, but, then, again, why is life expectancy in Puerto Rico over seventy-nine? Health spending and health policy are determined by elected officials. Elected officials are chosen by voters. If the grass appears greener on the other side of the state line, it's up to citizens to demand better care of their grass.

Finally, local politics are also important. Local, state, and federal representatives often vote based on feedback from constituents. Write letters, send emails, and make phone calls. Tell them what you think. Social media also has an important role to play here. A well-placed social media post can sometimes get much more attention from politicians than traditional methods ever could. Politicians usually have a lot of clout with hospitals as well. Furthermore, many hospitals are integral parts of the communities they serve. Hospitals have boards of directors or trustees, and most are from the local community. Most hospital trustees will tell you that they rarely if ever hear from the public. When our local hospital engages in unethical business practices like suing patients over unpaid medical bills, we should contact the hospitals trustees and ask why.

ABOUT THE AUTHOR

John A. Kellum, MD, is a distinguished professor of Critical Care Medicine and holds an endowed chair in Critical Care Research at the University of Pittsburgh. He has been a practicing intensive care physician for more than thirty years. His experience in hospital boardrooms and at ICU bedsides has informed the writing of this book, exposing the real dangers we are facing in American healthcare. Dangers which, almost inexplicably, are not being discussed at the national level even as they are whispered by physicians to one another in the corridors and break rooms of every hospital in the US.

Dr. Kellum received his medical degree from the Medical College of Ohio in 1984. His postgraduate training includes an internship and residency in Internal Medicine at the University of Rochester, New York, and a fellowship in Critical Care Medicine at the University of Pittsburgh. He is a highly cited researcher whose interests span various aspects of critical care medicine but center in critical care nephrology, sepsis, and multi-organ failure. He has authored more than 750 publications and has won several awards for teaching. He lectures widely and has given more than one thousand seminars and invited lectures worldwide.